Rima D. Apple
Janet Golden
Editors

Women and Prenatal Testing

Facing the Challenges of Genetic Technology

EDITED BY

Karen H. Rothenberg and
Elizabeth J. Thomson

Ohio State University Press

COLUMBUS

Library of Congress Cataloging-in-Publication Data

Women and prenatal testing : facing the challenges of genetic
    technology / edited by Karen H. Rothenberg and Elizabeth J. Thomson.
        p.   cm. — (Women and health)
    Includes bibliographical references.
    ISBN 0-8142-0640-9 (cloth : acid-free paper). — ISBN
0-8142-0641-7 (paper : acid-free paper)
        1. Prenatal diagnosis—Moral and ethical aspects.   2. Prenatal
diagnosis—Social aspects.   3. Prenatal diagnosis—Psychological
aspects.   I. Rothenberg, Karen H., 1952–   .   II. Thomson,
Elizabeth Jean.   III. Series: Women & health (Columbus, Ohio)
RG628.W65   1994
618.3′2042—dc20   94-6363
                                                                                    CIP

Text and jacket design by James F. Brisson.
Type set in Bembo by G&S Typesetters, Inc., Austin, Texas.
Printed by Bookcrafters, Chelsea, Michigan.

The paper in this book meets the guidelines for permanence
and durability of the Committee on Production Guidelines for
Book Longevity of the Council on Library Resources. ∞

9 8 7 6 5 4 3 2 1

This book is dedicated to our families,
Jeff, Andrea, and Becky Seltzer
and Jim and Jennifer Hanson,
with love.

CONTENTS

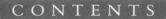

ACKNOWLEDGMENTS

The editors would like to thank Dr. Duane Alexander, Director of the National Institute of Child Health and Human Development (NICHD), and "Gil" (James G.) Hill, who was then Chief of the Office of Science Policy and Analysis at NICHD, for their support and encouragement in putting on the National Institutes of Health workshop, "Reproductive Genetic Testing: Impact on Women." It was this meeting that provided the stimulus for this book. Special thanks go to Dr. Eric Juengst, Chief of the Ethical, Legal, and Social Implications Branch of the National Center for Human Genome Research, for sharing his remarkable insights both during and after the meeting and for the center's support of this meeting. Thanks also go to the National Institute of Nursing Research and the Office of Research on Women's Health of the National Institutes of Health (NIH) for their contributions to this meeting.

We would also like to thank the participants of the NIH workshop. The interaction with the participants was an extremely powerful experience and influenced our thinking as well as the thinking of others who attended this meeting. In some ways these interactions forever changed how we and others perceive these issues.

A very special thank-you goes to secretaries Kathy Montroy and Mickey Hannah McCoy: Kathy for her many contributions, from typing portions of the manuscript, to following up with contributors to ensure they responded in a timely fashion; and Mickey for her help in organizing the workshop and communicating with participants both before and after the workshop.

Finally, we would like to express our everlasting gratitude to our families who have patiently supported us through the rigors of the workshop, this publication, and many other activities associated with our work. It is to our families that this book is dedicated.

Although we were once told that outer space was the next frontier, as the domain of knowledge about ourselves expands, our society's focus is instead turning inward, to the human body. In probing the human genome, we are learning not only about life, but about its meaning, as we are forced to explore the implication of the new research agenda. What will it mean to know about the genetics of a fetus? Who will control the production of this new knowledge? Who will interpret its meaning? Who will decide what actions need to be taken?

Questions such as these led to the convening of a conference on women and the Human Genome Project in November, 1991, and eventually to the preparation of this volume of essays. The editors have woven together the diverse voices of scholars, from humanists to social researchers. Together, they seek to understand what prenatal genetic testing means for women today and what its ramifications are for the future. These scholars have not given us a road map, but instead a traveler's guide to warn of the challenges we face as we journey to this new territory. All of us—students and academics, patients and professionals, voters and public servants—will have to consider carefully the implications of prenatal genetic testing.

We are particularly pleased to have this volume in our Women and Health series because of its multifaceted approach to highly controversial issues. The book raises significant questions for a society challenged by new technologies and new experiences. The authors demand that we promote an environment in which women's voices are incorporated into the debate. It is a demand that must be heard.

I met Molly in the spring of 1991 at the time that Karen and I were organizing the National Institutes of Health meeting, "Reproductive Genetic Testing: Impact on Women." Molly was in a state of desperation. She was six weeks pregnant and was scheduled to have her pregnancy terminated, but she did not want the abortion—she wanted a baby. A mutual friend asked if I would be willing to talk with her because he knew that I had been an obstetrics nurse and then a genetics counselor for the past 20 years. From our first phone conversation it was clear that the story of Molly's pregnancy demonstrated many of the anticipated and unanticipated effects of today's ongoing developments in reproductive genetic testing on women. Her experience further strengthened our commitment to discover the many social, medical, and ethical issues that need to be addressed as these technologies unfold.

Molly's pregnancy was one entirely planned and very much desired. She had had a problem with infertility, and this pregnancy had been conceived while taking a fertility drug. Immediately after conception the tests had begun, and they were repeated on a weekly basis. Through weekly ultrasound and hormone examinations, her doctor determined that her hormone level was low and that the embryo was "lagging one week behind in 'its' growth."

After I first spoke with her, I called a colleague of mine from the Midwest. She agreed with me that although the findings were worrisome, they probably didn't support any perceived sense of urgency on the part of Molly's provider to terminate a desired pregnancy. It was possible too, we thought, that her pregnancy was one destined to spontaneously abort. We agreed that one approach Molly might consider was a conservative one, to wait a little longer to see what would happen.

Molly and I had dinner together on a Tuesday. She seemed troubled, tired, and at times distraught. I told her the little that I knew—and of the many things I didn't. I encouraged her to talk with her provider, to ask a number of questions before her scheduled abortion, which was to take place on Thursday. At times she cried. I asked her again whether she wanted the abortion, and she said no. She could ask the physician, I suggested, what would happen if they waited a week or two. She hadn't realized that that was an option. I told her that poor growth in the embryo along with a low hormone level could be an indication that she would have a miscarriage. While a miscarriage, of course, does not make a pregnancy loss any less painful, in Molly's case the circumstances of the loss seemed preferable to intentional termination.

The next day she visited her physician. After many questions and a long discussion, the abortion was postponed—not canceled, but postponed. He said they would watch and wait for another week and then repeat the tests again. A week later the tests revealed that the embryo was continuing to lag a week behind in growth, and the hormone level continued to be low. The abortion was rescheduled for the following week. When I spoke with Molly again, she was beside herself. She was terribly concerned about her baby, but she still wasn't convinced by the test results that her pregnancy should be terminated. She decided that she wanted a second opinion, and one was arranged by her provider.

The second opinion, however, resulted in confusing information, leaving Molly wondering what to believe. Concerns had been expressed about Molly's mental health and well-being as a result of this pregnancy. I questioned whether her well-being was jeopardized, not by the pregnancy, but by all that had gone on during her pregnancy. Molly had already been through so much, and she was only eight weeks pregnant.

Soon thereafter, Molly saw an obstetrician. She remarked to me that the obstetrician seemed to treat her and her baby quite differently than had her infertility specialist. Although I am unsure of the significance of her observation, similar observations have been verbalized to me by women in similar circumstances. Nonetheless, the weekly ultrasound and hormone evaluations stopped. She stopped being an infertile woman seeing an infertility specialist and started being a pregnant woman receiving prenatal care.

Three weeks went by, nothing happened, and Molly was feeling better. No one had checked the size of her baby by ultrasound or monitored her hormone levels during that time. But now it was time for her chorionic villi sampling. I spoke with her about the procedure, and she seemed to have a fairly good understanding of the physical risks associated with the procedure. She also knew they would be looking for chromosome abnormalities such as that seen in Down syndrome. She was over 40 and, from most people's perspective, checking for chromosome abnormalities seemed to be the standard thing to do.

The procedure went well; there were no complications. Two weeks later she called: It was a boy! He had 46 chromosomes, and she only had 28 weeks to go. I was delighted by her news, but I couldn't help having nagging concerns that something undetectable in the chromosomes could still be wrong. I certainly didn't want to convey my worries to Molly, though; she had enough worries of her own.

Three more weeks went by, and it was time for Molly's maternal serum alpha-fetoprotein screening (MSAFP) test. The chorionic villi sampling test isn't capable of detecting open spine defects, and MSAFP is the test done to attempt to ensure the absence of this defect. The next time Molly called, she was upset again. The MSAFP test result was abnormal, and she wanted to know what that could mean. She had talked to her obstetrician who indicated that the baby's spine might be open, and she was scheduled to have an amniocentesis to clarify the meaning of this apparently "abnormal" result. Trying to think through all of her options, we discussed the various reasons that the MSAFP might be elevated, including the possibility of normal human variation—something no one else had mentioned to her.

The amniocentesis procedure went well, with no accompanying complications, but the results were puzzling: No clear explanation had been found for the MSAFP elevation. There didn't appear to be an open spine defect, but the amniotic fluid–AFP level was also elevated. There seemed to be no explanation for this finding either. A few days later Molly got a call from her physician. A mistake had been made: The calculations done to obtain the result on her amniotic fluid–AFP level had been done incorrectly. The results of the amniocentesis AFP level were normal. Molly cried. She called me, and she cried.

The rest of Molly's pregnancy was, to everyone's relief, medically uneventful. I remember my own nagging concerns for Molly and her expected baby. There had been so many times when I wondered whether he would ever make it. And there had even been times when I wondered whether Molly would make it. Tommy was born in November of 1991. Tommy is now two, he's healthy, and Molly is thinking of having another baby.

While Molly's story may be viewed as anecdotal, it is a true story and one that illustrates a number of the issues raised by the increasing use and "routinization" of prenatal diagnostic tests. Some, if not all, parts of this story have been chronicled by other women and substantiated by many other providers of genetic services. This is not an isolated incident, nor is it an uncommon story. It is, however, one that documents the very necessity of our facing the broader implications of these developing technologies. Such stories remind us that these tests are not only medical procedures; they are intimately connected with women's lives. Moreover, such stories and the analyses that follow challenge us to look beyond the narrow confines of medical and research settings and to further anticipate and begin to understand the broader effects of reproductive genetic testing on women, their relationships, and their pregnancy experiences.

Elizabeth J. Thomson

The names in this account have been changed to protect the privacy of those involved.

Women and Prenatal Testing:

An Introduction to the Issues

KAREN H. ROTHENBERG AND
ELIZABETH J. THOMSON

Childbearing in the 1990s has brought with it new and expanding reproductive genetic testing options. These developments have led some to claim that now is an ideal time to be having children because the new procedures provide women with previously unavailable information about their pregnancies. Others maintain, however, that in the era prior to the advent of these options, reproductive ignorance was bliss. They contend that with fewer diagnostic interventions, fewer reproductive decisions were required of women. Today, some would claim that this increasing knowledge mandates increasing and perhaps unwarranted responsibility. While some women have greater knowledge about their pregnancies, so too do they face increasing pressure to do as much as is technologically possible to ensure the birth of a healthy child.

Along with these reproductive testing options have come obstacles that create new challenges. Reproductive genetic technologies are complex and difficult for many women to comprehend. Their purposes, benefits, risks, and limitations are not uniformly defined by providers nor fully understood by many women. Today, prenatal testing can disclose hundreds of disorders. Treatment or cure, however, is not possible for most of them. Some providers state that prenatal and perinatal care can sometimes be improved through increased prenatal knowledge. Yet in many cases there is nothing that can be done to improve

1

the outcome of the pregnancy, other than to terminate the pregnancy or prepare for the birth of a child with a disability.

In the majority of cases, especially when the disorder is perceived as serious, women choose to terminate the pregnancy. Some providers of reproductive genetic testing services do not provide the abortion services and, as a result, many women feel isolated and abandoned at this time in their pregnancy. Clearly, prenatal genetic knowledge does not necessarily guarantee successful treatment, cure, or care. Yet despite the lack of treatment or cure for diagnosed conditions, more women are being offered these services. Many women feel obliged to accept testing; they do not perceive that they have a choice. Ironically, many other women, because of little or no access to prenatal care, are also denied reproductive genetic testing services, even when they are desired.

As reproductive genetic technologies expand and provide more information about genetic diversity, so too does the complexity increase of the issues raised. For example, some proponents of first trimester prenatal diagnostic methods such as chorionic villi sampling (CVS) contend that early diagnosis will result in better care for women, especially for those in whose expected child a birth defect or genetic disorder is identified. Women who face the decision about whether to continue or terminate a pregnancy would thereby be allowed to make the decision in the first trimester rather than in the second. Although anecdotal reports exist, there is no scientific evidence supporting the assumption that first trimester fetal diagnosis actually makes prenatal diagnosis better for women. Whereas evidence exists that pregnancy termination is biologically safer in the first trimester, there is no corresponding evidence that it is psychologically easier. It may also be true that natural pregnancy loss would have resulted in a number of cases in which a genetic disorder was identified early and the pregnancy was intentionally terminated. Thus, it should be considered that one result of earlier prenatal testing may in fact yield a larger number of women faced with the decision of whether to continue or terminate a pregnancy. Additionally, because CVS does not provide information about one of the most common birth defects (spina bifida and other neural tube defects), women will be encouraged to undergo further testing for these conditions into the second trimester of pregnancy. What impact does such periodic testing have on women and their pregnancy experiences?

Advocates for the development of the noninvasive methods of prenatal diagnostic methods believe that eliminating the potential biological risks associated with prenatal testing will make the decision to have prenatal testing easier for women. Whether the development of noninvasive methods for prenatal testing will make women's decisions to have prenatal diagnosis more or less complicated is not known. Will there be some risk for increased directiveness on the part of providers to ensure that the testing is carried out? Will such noninvasive testing be moved further into the realm of routine testing that is carried out as a part of prenatal care? Will women feel even more obliged to accept testing when there are no biological risks associated with the procedure?

In order to begin responding to some of these issues, a workshop was held in the fall of 1991 on the campus of the National Institutes of Health. This meeting was cosponsored by the National Institute of Child Health and Human Development, the National Center for Human Genome Research, the National Center for Nursing Research, and the Office of Research on Women's Health. It was designed to provide a forum for dialogue among the basic scientists, providers of these services, social scientists, ethicists, and lawyers on how best to begin to address these issues. At the end of this book, in the appendix, is the Workshop Summary Statement highlighting some of the themes that emerged from the discussions of that meeting. The proceedings of the entire workshop were published in the journal, *Fetal Diagnosis and Therapy* (1993) Vol. 8, Suppl. 1.

This book is designed to focus primarily on the major women's issues surrounding the development and application of reproductive genetic testing. Although the literature is filled with articles addressing the biological safety and efficacy of these technologies, only a small amount of literature is devoted to the psychological, sociocultural, ethical, legal, or political impact of their application on women and their pregnancy experience. Following this brief introduction is a series of chapters designed to stimulate discussion on the complex issues being raised by the increasing application of prenatal genetic technologies. Featured are the voices and questions of women coming from a variety of perspectives and experiences. A number of the authors have themselves been consumers of such services.

The book is divided into three main parts: The Context of Debate; Philosophical, Ethical, and Legal Perspectives; and Psychological and Sociocultural Issues. Part 1 provides the contextual framework through which the debate should be analyzed. Part 2 sets forth the philosophical foundations and complex ethical questions raised, as well as the types of legal issues that need to be addressed. Part 3 delineates a variety of perspectives on pertinent psychological and sociocultural issues.

Our goal is to examine reproductive genetic testing in the context of women's lives. Potentially, the major risk associated with reproductive genetic testing may come in not knowing how to cope with the information obtained from these procedures, rather than with the procedures themselves. Such knowledge may have a lasting impact on women, their families, and their pregnancy experiences. These and other issues will need to continue to be addressed in order to confirm or deny the anticipated benefits and risks of developing reproductive genetic technologies. It is our intention that this book will contribute to a further understanding of the issues.

The Context of Debate

The three chapters in this part provide the contextual framework through which the debate on the complex issues raised by reproductive genetic testing should be analyzed. Abby Lippman argues that the application of prenatal genetic testing both reflects and generates the process of "geneticization" that increasingly orients contemporary stories of health and disease in our Western culture. She examines some of the stories being told about prenatal testing and questions their themes of reassurance and choice, their construction of risk, and their assumptions about disability. She explores the lifestyle testing creates for pregnant women, the testing itself, and its power to control both how we live and the children we bear. Complex and troubling questions are brought to the light that require examination: Would women naturally be concerned about these genetic risk factors during pregnancy if those risk factors weren't sought out and identified by health care providers? Do women subsequently have their heightened anxiety relieved, sometimes falsely so, when the results of the testing provided turn out to be normal?

With this contextual framework in place, Ruth Schwartz Cowan provides a historical perspective on two commonly used prenatal procedures: amniocentesis and chorionic villi sampling. This history indicates that women have played differing roles in the developmental and diffusion stages of both pro-

cedures. Effective future policies regarding the impact of prenatal diagnosis on women may be shaped by lessons learned
from that history. Based on such a perspective, how might
women have a greater impact on defining the future directions
of developing technologies based on their actual needs and
interests?

Increasing attention focused on the development and utilization of prenatal testing may have the risk of further stigmatizing
individuals with disabilities. Deborah Kaplan examines and describes policy implications of prenatal testing with those concerns in mind. She argues that the most troubling and controversial aspect of prenatal testing is when it results in selective
abortion. The most common reasons cited for selective abortion due to disability are based on assumptions made about persons with disabilities, most of which have been neither confirmed nor refuted by research. Is there a known and predictable
quality of life that is associated with specific birth defects or
genetic disorders? By whose standard should an individual's
quality of life be judged? Is life with a disability worse than no
life at all? What potential impact does the increasing availability
of prenatal testing have on public attitudes about disability and
practices toward people with disabilities?

1

The Genetic Construction
of Prenatal Testing:

Choice, Consent, or Conformity
for Women?

ABBY LIPPMAN

Biomedical researchers are currently redefining human geography. These modern explorers are elaborat-
ing a new human map, based on genes, that is likely to alter
our views of the world—and our place in it—even more profoundly than did the maps generated by Columbus and other
fifteenth- and sixteenth-century explorers. More important,
this newest expression of territorial expansion and colonization, a process I call geneticization and describe more fully below, is likely also to alter our perceptions of self and other, of
normality and abnormality, particularly in the area of procreation. This can be seen most clearly in the consideration of the
impacts of prenatal genetic testing and screening on women.

The application of prenatal genetic screening and testing—
and I use the terms generically, if imprecisely, to encompass the
range of activities from amniocentesis through ultrasound to
embryo analysis—raises a number of fundamental concerns related to women's health and health care simply because they are
techniques applied to women. How, when, why, and to and by
whom they are applied will be conditioned by prevailing attitudes about women, their bodies, and their roles. Although
some concerns pertain especially to only certain groups of
women, those that I will emphasize cut across color, ability,
economic, and sexual orientation lines and are relevant to all
women. Being developed in a world that is gendered, the ge-

netic and other reproductive technologies cannot escape gendered use, use that reflects prevalent ideas about women.[1] Thus,
even if the technologies have not been developed and used specifically to maintain gendered distinctions and increase patriarchal power, as some have suggested (Rowland, 1984), prenatal testing cannot be considered as neutral in North America
or any other society in which inequality exists between the
sexes. Women remain politically and economically disadvantaged, have limited access to services, and are continually
challenged by prejudicial norms surrounding motherhood, in
addition to being delegated responsibility for family health.
Women experience testing, therefore, not merely as parents, but
as mothers. Applying prenatal technologies, when disability in
a child is viewed as a private problem for a family, is not only
a matter of testing a parent who will care for a child, but of
examining the woman who is to be a mother responsible for
avoiding, reducing, or managing disability in her offspring.

Let me emphasize that I am working under the assumption
that prenatal testing is problematic for all women, users and
nonusers, supporters and critics alike. In no way do I intend my
remarks about it to reflect negatively on women who have considered or undergone testing; criticism of the technologies is not
criticism of them. Women considering childbearing today face
agonizing issues that I was fortunate enough not to have to confront, and as I learn from them I can only admire and respect
their tremendous strength and resilience.

Background of Prenatal Genetic Testing

When first developed, prenatal diagnosis was employed for
conditions generally regarded by physicians as serious and for
which there were no treatments. It is now available for conditions with little or uncertain impact on postnatal health and
functioning, conditions that will appear—if at all—only in
adulthood, and conditions for which effective treatments exist.
Clearly, the number of complications that can be discovered
with prenatal testing is expanding: the earliest time period when
attempts to detect problems are made is being moved back from
the 14–20 week period when amniocentesis is employed to the

10–12 week slot allotted to chorionic villi sampling (CVS). Indeed, a woman need not even be pregnant now to obtain "prenatal" diagnosis because embryos procured following in vitro fertilization can be examined before they are implanted.

The expansions being made in the definitions of the categories of subjects, objects, and timing of prenatal diagnosis are troubling. But even without those issues, many thousands of women, pregnant or not, are already confronted by the need to consider how much, if at all, they want to know about a fetus during pregnancy, what wanting or not wanting this information entails and implies, and how they feel about disability. The very availability of those technologies necessarily forces every woman at least to consider if she desires genetic testing—or if she even desires that testing be available for use by other women—and merely facing this choice is itself difficult, and often painful (cf. Lippman-Hand & Fraser, 1979a, 1979b).

Prenatal genetic testing is not just another improvement in obstetric care, despite the tendency of some to call it routine, or even banal (Dumez, 1989). Rather, deciding for or against testing makes many women feel they will be making a terrible mistake regardless of the path chosen. With the application of genetic testing earlier and earlier in fetal life, and with the growing number of variations now detectable (some of which may only increase susceptibility to the later development of a treatable medical problem), it seems urgent that we directly examine the real reasons we are testing women and fetuses, what it means to test them, how testing establishes boundaries for what we call normal, and how changes in us, our relationships, and the children we bear may be embedded in testing. To start this examination it is useful to look at some of the stories told about health, disease, and prenatal testing.

Stories and Storytellers

In our contemporary Western culture, we tend to cling to the seemingly unproblematic belief that the pursuit of biomedical knowledge of health and disease is a sign of progress. We all too often forget that despite their biological reality, human diseases, disorders, and disabilities—the objects of prenatal screening—

are not just physical or physiological states with fixed contours. Rather than merely being "out there" awaiting our discovery, they are social products with variable shapes and distributions that we fashion, interpret, and give meaning to via our beliefs, attitudes, values, and interests. Western biomedicine is our ethnomedicine, and it does not describe a preexisting biological reality. Particular social and cultural assumptions (Wright & Treacher, 1982) influence the scientific researchers who give the biological processes of observed diseases particular forms through their diagnostic labels and causal attributions. Those forms vary across different human groups and at different periods of time. How the processes are counted, defined, and studied, and how people are assigned to the categories created, is necessarily context-specific, reflecting how those with power at any particular historical time construct a particular physiological or physical condition as a problem. These constructions are what I call "stories."

By using the word story I do not intend to suggest that what is said or written about health and disease is not true. This may or may not be the case, but that discussion is not relevant here. I use the word in a literary rather than a legal sense to capture the idea that scientists choose their subject matter and present their observations, their research, in the same way as novelists select some arbitrary slice of life to describe and interpret the external world. Both groups, both sets of authors, shape and interpret raw material to convey a message, reducing its complexity in order to tell a story. Their constructions reflect their personal views and the prevailing political, social, and cultural context.

Because the distribution of health and disease is influenced by many factors—social and physical environments, economic conditions, gender, racial identity, personal behaviors, and available health services, as well as heredity—biomedical scientists have a wealth of raw material from which to choose when they construct their explanations, their stories, for the conditions that interest them. The factors they choose to (re)create stories and metaphors about health and disease, and the subsequent expression of those choices in public policies and private practices, will reflect the background beliefs, the vested interests, and the ideologies of both those studying such matters and those funding their studies.

Stories, in general, rearrange that which is complex into shapes that simplify and tame. This certainly characterizes the stories about health and disease in today's professional and popular media that are being told increasingly in the language of genetics. Using the metaphor of blueprints, with genes and DNA fragments presented as a set of instructions, the dominant discourse describing the human condition is reductionist, emphasizing a genetic determination for our various frailties and differences from one another, with the double helix employed as illustrative icon (Myers, 1990). In standard Cartesian tradition the body is viewed as a machine comprising replaceable parts, with genes and DNA sequences being the essential components of these parts. The author of a recent book about genetics selected for distribution by the Book-of-the-Month Club may have been extreme in enthusiastically describing human diseases as "typographical errors" (Shapiro, 1990), but his narrative was not out of line with today's best-selling stories telling how increased understanding of disease and the improvement of health can only be produced by studying (and mapping) genes and developing tests to establish our, and our children's, genetic status and chemical individuality.

I use the term "geneticization" to capture this single conceptual model that is increasingly elicited to reveal and explain health and disease, normality and abnormality, and that is directing the application of intellectual and financial resources for resolving health problems, profoundly affecting our values and attitudes (Lippman, 1991; Lippman, Messing, & Mayer, 1990). Geneticization refers to the ongoing process by which priority is given to searching for variations in DNA sequences that differentiate people from each other and to attributing some hereditary basis to most disorders, behaviors, and physiological variations (including such things as schizophrenia and high blood pressure as well as the ability of children to sit still while watching television and of adults to quit smoking). Whereas "energetic physicians" once "discerned microorganisms responsible for almost every ill known to mankind [sic]" (Rosenberg, 1992), their latter-day heirs discern genes. In this sense, geneti-

cization is a process of colonization with genetic technologies
and approaches applied to areas not necessarily—or even apparently—genetic.

As geneticization becomes an ever louder theme in stories of
health and disease, prenatal genetic screening and testing take
on major roles in the search to find those who have certain genetic differences thought to be associated with what is considered biomedically abnormal. Indeed, applying these technologies increases the numbers of those with conditions labeled as
genetic or with variations called abnormal, and establishes hi-
erarchies among individuals based on their sought-after DNA
differences. Carried out on women who experience unequal distributions of health that reflect class, race, and other social strati-
fications in North America, prenatal genetic screening and testing technologies have a vast shaping power likely to reinforce
existing standards and power relationships. This alone makes
an examination of those stories especially appropriate.

Stories about Prenatal Testing

As a major component of genetic stories of health and disease,
prenatal diagnosis is given its own narrative shape. Attractively
phrased, medically oriented arguments provide the key motifs
in reports of prenatal testing, reports that serve largely to natu-
ralize the activity by shaping it as a means for "reproductive
autonomy," a way of giving women information that will expand their reproductive choices (Lippman, 1986). As such, it is
stated to be a response to the "needs" of pregnant women for
reassurance, something women "choose." (A subtext in contemporary biomedical stories about prenatal diagnosis presents
it as a public health activity to reduce the frequency of selected
birth defects, but this theme is usually considerably muted for
reasons discussed elsewhere [Lippman, 1986, 1989]).

Unfortunately, the dominant (need/choice) presentation is
incomplete because it fails to capture the internal tension of
prenatal genetic testing. This tension arises because testing
comprises at least two sets of conflicting activities. As supporters claim, it may be a way to give women some control over
their pregnancies, respecting (and increasing) their autonomy to

choose the kinds of children they will bear (Hill, 1986). It may be a means of reassuring women that could enhance their experience of pregnancy (Royal College of Physicians, 1989) by providing a way to avoid the family distress and suffering associated with the unpredicted birth of babies with genetic disorders or congenital malformations. But, as critics claim, it is also an assembly line approach to the products of conception, separating out those products we wish to develop from those we wish to discontinue (Ewing, 1990; Rothman, 1989)—though biomedical authors continually reject any suggestion that testing may be eugenic.

The language of control, choice, and reassurance used by supporters, usually biomedical authors, certainly makes prenatal diagnosis appear attractive and is, at first reading, persuasive. (This discourse is also more likely to succeed as a colonizing strategy than one employing an image of selection.) But in reading the pleasing biomedical stories closely, several problems (beyond those of the absence of good empiric evidence to support the claim that control, autonomy, and reassurance are actually enhanced) are brought to the light.

First, these are but partial stories because they exclude the words of women who ignore their physicians' urgings for amniocentesis and reject testing in order not to lose the assurances provided by their own bodies that they are healthy and normal. One particularly eloquent teller of such a story explained that she sought reassurance from what concerned her by refusing testing when pregnant at age 38. She perceived her risk as a pregnant woman not in terms of having a child with Down syndrome, but in terms of what might ensue if she entered a process of medical surveillance. She feared testing would enmesh her in a system that would produce problems and create experiences likely to undermine her pleasure of pregnancy, and she didn't want to divert her energy from enjoying her pregnancy to fighting this system. Her story is not unique, and for a more complete description we need to situate prenatal testing and grapple with its contradictions; we must include such experiences told by women in their own ways. Reassurance comes from many sources, not all of which are linked to genetic testing.

Second, to tell the story of prenatal testing univocally, in the language of reassurance, is clearly too simplistic. Notwithstanding that genetic testing can be selectively reassuring for the vast majority of women in prenatal diagnosis programs who will learn that their fetuses do not have Down syndrome, the bold text offers rhetorical camouflage and evades questions about why reassurance is sought, how its provision is circumscribed, and how prenatal testing may actually threaten women's well-being and create dis-ease. It hides the iatrogenic nature of "need" by failing to ask whether reassurance would be sought if an outsider had not first decided that certain women were at risk and that the condition for which the risk existed warranted diagnosis before a baby with it was born. It hides the need to consider the possibility that reassurance is a biomedical fix disempowering women and increasing their dependency on technology.

The concept of risk dominates the process of becoming a mother in North America today (Quéniart, 1988). Women are categorized from the time of a first prenatal visit into high- and low-risk groups, with membership in a "no-risk" group possible only in retrospect. By attaching a risk label to pregnancy, physicians reconstruct a normal experience, making it one that requires their supervision. This becomes especially clear in the context of the major application of prenatal genetic testing to date: here risk has been conceptualized strictly in terms of a woman's age, with those 35 years and older automatically and homogeneously labeled as belonging to a high-risk group warranting prenatal diagnosis because of their statistical probability of giving birth to a child with Down syndrome. While presented as a biomedical fact, however, this recommendation is actually more a social statement about the status of the woman and the quality of her fetus. For example, despite the biomedical classification, women 35 and older are not the only ones at risk for having a child with Down syndrome. In addition, the discontinuity imposed by this particular age cutoff is medically arbitrary, since the probability of fetal chromosome abnormality increases smoothly with a woman's age (Vekemans & Lippman, 1984). All women have some risk of having a child with Down syndrome. What defines one probability as high and another as low?

The location of a statistical boundary to separate high- or low-risk groups is historically and politically contingent. In France, for example, "risk" apparently begins only at 38 years, since this is when public funds first cover services (Moatti et al., 1989). Age 35 as the point of entry to a genetic risk group and as the criterion for prenatal testing probably replaced the initial threshold in North America—which was no less arbitrarily set at age 40—in response to cost-benefit analyses and service needs assessments undertaken as prenatal diagnosis was developed.[2] Certainly, no new information was produced to indicate that women ages 35 to 39 were at greater risk than they had been a decade earlier when 40 was the magic threshold. Nor had women's biology changed. Rather, definitions and expectations of normal pregnancies intersected with developments in prenatal diagnosis and a growing "ideology of risk" surrounding pregnancy; the worries about Down syndrome and the quest for normal offspring turned into technical problems to be overcome, with prenatal testing being the response. The process, we should note, continues today with proposals to further lower, if not remove, the age limit for amniocentesis proliferating. Getting "older," it seems, is getting younger every day (Hubbard, 1984). And with more and more women being told that their age (thus, in effect *they*) create a risk for the fetus, the number wanting reassurance through testing to allay iatrogenic worries can only increase.

Moreover, having a prenatal screening test specifically oriented to detect a particular condition—and Down syndrome provides a compelling example—expresses a social statement about the quality or the value of fetuses and children based solely on their genetic or chromosomal material. Through these programs we are saying it is okay if children with certain chromosomes are not born, and that having the condition detected is, in effect, worse than being alive (Asch, 1988). And we underscore this by invariably considering the abortion of a fetus with some disorder as a core benefit, not a worrisome cost (Clarke, in press), when economic analyses of screening programs are carried out.

Further, the power to set boundaries for who may or may not be born remains with those university researchers and for-profit laboratories who develop and deploy the technologies of

testing. Only the conditions for which they make tests available
can be sought, with what is available determined by their agendas for professional recognition or financial profit—by their social values. Here, as elsewhere, individuals may seem to choose,
but it is only from options constrained by the limitations of
possibilities created by others (Lippman, 1989).

Thus, for a complete understanding of how reassurance relates to prenatal testing programs for women 35 and older and
to their acceptance of these procedures, we need to situate the
biomedical stories in the historical and cultural context in which
notions of risk and attitudes toward normality are constructed.
When we remember that in North America today, pregnancy
has largely come to be seen as baby production (Martin, 1987)
with the laborer, the pregnant woman who will produce the
baby, being held to certain standards (Rothman, 1989), it is not
unreasonable to call stories about testing incomplete if they fail
to take into account its use to ensure the quality of both mother
and child. Prenatal testing provides "reassuring" quality control and consumer protection, necessarily involving system-
atic and systemic selection of fetuses, most frequently on genetic grounds. Biomedicine can't directly change the risk to the
quality of the "product" stemming from a woman's age, the
probability of chromosomal nondisjunction leading to Down
syndrome. But rereading the reassurance text reveals that biomedicine claims it will control its *impact* by providing testing
to identify "products" of lesser quality—fetuses with Down
syndrome—and prevent the birth of those that are "abnormal."
If, then, reassurance is produced following prenatal diagnosis,
it is, at best, an acquired rather than inherent characteristic of
testing, tranquilizing women who have first been made fearful.

So, before screening or testing for Down syndrome is further
extended to reassure women of all chronological ages, let us
reclaim the term and consider alternative stories about reassurance that respond to the desire of all pregnant women for
healthy children and do not rely on prenatal testing and genetic
control. For instance, the unacceptably large number of pregnant women living below the poverty line would probably like
reassurance that their babies could develop as well as the babies
of wealthier women and not be at increased risk for the childhood mortality and morbidity associated with low birth weight

and prematurity. Why not reassure them by providing the adequate diet required to prevent low birth weight? Why not allocate public funds for home visitors, respite care, and domestic alterations that would permit women to manage their special needs should their children be born with (or as is more likely, later develop), a health problem? These and other alternative approaches would provide reassurance to many women, would provide this reassurance with respect to (and for) fetal disability, and would diminish a woman's feeling of personal responsibility for a child's health (Farrant, 1985). Furthermore, they would not require women to select fetuses based on their characteristics.

Stories about prenatal testing that imply that the testing is really only a response to the needs of pregnant women for reassurance, something women choose, may seem sensible in a society that still allocates major responsibility for family health care to women and assumes that they must do all that is recommended or available to foster their children's health. But is there really choice? Is a full range of options truly available? Continuing a pregnancy when the fetus has been found to have Down syndrome cannot be considered a real option when society does not truly accept children with disabilities or provide assistance for their nurturance (cf. Retsinas, 1991). It is not surprising that a woman offered ultrasound by an expert—who implies that she really wants to have a healthy child, doesn't she?—perceives a need to be tested, a need to do all that is recommended (for her peace of mind, if nothing else). Is her agreement, then, to testing an expression of choice or an instance of conformity? When prenatal testing is presented as giving nature a helping hand because most fetuses with malformations are spontaneously aborted (for example, about 80% of fetuses with Down syndrome), is induced abortion perceived as a choice or as an automatic (natural) component of testing? And when those of us who are not pregnant repeatedly hear or read stories about the increasing frequency of genetic disorders and their further strain on already overextended medical systems, how can supporting the extension of testing programs not seem an appropriate social "choice" to deal with this so-called public health problem (Rowland, 1984).[3]

To no one's surprise, a woman may need some extra help to

raise a child with a disability. If society does not respect and meet her needs appropriately, she will, as is understandable, seek a way to avoid the problem. If prenatal testing and abortion of fetuses with the disability constitute the only solution offered, a need for screening gets created. But without real options that respect a woman for herself, not for her role as producer, choice may be a misnomer.

Legitimate efforts to avoid unnecessary harm to a fetus or a woman in a continuing pregnancy and to protect both from avoidable death or disability are essential. But if healthy children really matter to us, as we say they do, is prenatal testing the best way to express our concern? All—or even most—that interferes with this idealized health status is not obviously genetic. And if healthy children really matter to us, their mothers must matter first. The well-being of children and the well-being of women are inseparable. Social, political, and economic neglect of women interferes with the physical and mental development of their children more than does the genetic variation they inherit. The physical violence experienced by 10% of women during their pregnancies cannot but affect their children's health too. If we value the mother and not only the birth of a healthy child, we must attend to this violence and neglect and not just attend to their genes. To ensure a woman's agency, we must create the conditions in which agency can be fully exercised without limits on her options.

Thus, we should resist relying on prenatal genetic testing to ensure our children's health when employing it threatens to displace attention from society's role in creating illness and seriously risks women's general well-being. Prenatal genetic testing, already called a ritual for (white, middle-class) women older than 35 (Rapp, 1988), may actually threaten women's well-being with the circumstances of its use making it resemble an addiction: the practice is socially determined, it satisfies a need to feel good with a fix, it creates dependency, and it provides substitute gratification. Evidence of this addiction appears in stories that describe testing as a way to release a woman to enjoy her pregnancy, high with the reassurance that the fetus does not have Down syndrome. It appears when women come to depend on testing because they are told it will provide a healthy baby. And it appears in the photograph or videotape of her ultrasound scan proudly displayed by a pregnant woman that functions as a technological substitute for the changes in her body and feelings that might once have satisfied her about her pregnancy. Extending the parallel just a bit further suggests that regulation of prenatal testing will not preclude the dependence on technology that disempowers women any more than the regulation of drugs will preclude addiction. Detoxification requires a change in the circumstances that present use (of drugs and of testing) as a solution, especially when the technology (as drug use) creates a "lifestyle" among and for users that is troublesome.

Prenatal Testing as "Lifestyle"

Prenatal genetic testing creates a lifestyle for pregnant women to the extent that the use, if not the mere availability, of the technology inevitably shapes the experiences of maternity and, in some ways, even becomes an end in itself. Prenatal testing, like other technologies, creates a lifestyle because it shapes issues in new ways, translates everyday life, transforms definitions of natural, and determines how pregnant women ought to live. For example, data from ongoing studies by myself and others (Green, Statham, & Snowdon, 1992; Press & Browner, 1993) indicate that having all the prenatal tests offered, along with giving up alcohol and smoking, going to prenatal classes, and eating properly have already become established behaviors that "responsible" (white, middle-class) women say they do "for the baby's good" once pregnancy begins (cf. Green et al., 1992). In addition, the mere possibility that women can avoid the birth of a child with some malformation makes the occurrence of such a birth "regrettable" and not just unfortunate.

Further transformations result from other features intrinsic to the use and experience of prenatal testing:

1. Most obvious, and as Beeson (1984) first showed, prenatal testing shapes the experience and progression of pregnancy. It divides what is unique, and unitary, into two not always compatible experiences—a social pregnancy and a biological pregnancy—and requires a woman to adapt to the testing process

and to a physician's schedule. When she tells others about her pregnancy, when she visits her physician, where she receives her care, and what she acknowledges as evidence that things are going well all occur on "testing time" rather than "women's time" (Beeson, 1984). Rothman's term, the "tentative pregnancy," captures some of that notion (Rothman, 1986).

Moreover, because prenatal screening and diagnosis have come to be seen by providers as part of the taken-for-granted package of services for pregnant women, part of the lifestyle of maternity, the normative has been inverted; only women who *decline* screening are referred for genetic counseling in some jurisdictions (Green et al., 1992); only women who *reject* parts of the antenatal care package (if they are white and well-educated) are treated as somehow abnormal. There seems to be more room for maneuver for African-American and Asian-American women, interestingly enough, perhaps because their rejection of testing is taken (ethnocentrically?) as an expression of "difference" (cf. Clarke, in press).

2. Prenatal testing, by another process of division, separates a single entity, a pregnant woman, into two: herself and her fetus. And by shaping the fetus as separate and separable from the woman, an opportunity is provided to assign independent interests (and/or rights) to it—interests not just attached through the mother. Suddenly "fetal abuse" becomes a thinkable concept, and a pregnant woman can be subjected to rules, regulations, and duties established by those seeking to protect fetal interests. With this division, a responsible mother becomes one who does everything—takes all tests—to ensure fetal health (Robertson, 1983; Shaw, 1980). So while a woman may have no control over or responsibility for the chromosomal occurrence of Down syndrome, she can control the birth of a child with this condition by being tested. Thus, if a child with Down syndrome is born to a woman who has refused testing, this becomes an event for which the child's mother is responsible because she could have prevented its occurrence. The individual is made into an agent of the state. This is made explicit when a 38-year-old gives birth to a baby with Down syndrome and several professionals ask: Why didn't she get tested (Thomson, personal communication, 1992)? Given that prevention is in-

creasingly the goal of biomedicine, with what speed will the disabilities and variations that *can* be prevented because prenatal tests for them exist become those that *should* be prevented, with testing thereby reshaping eugenics into a private process of "selection by prevention" (Kuitert, 1988)?

3. Prenatal testing as a lifestyle shapes general attitudes toward disability in multiple ways. Most generally, testing presents disability as if it were simply a medical problem, hides the social roots of handicaps, and distracts attention from prevailing social, economic, and political policies whose failure to account for a wide distribution of abilities convert impairments into handicaps. Testing reshapes the problem of disability so that it need not be *ours* collectively to solve (what will *we* do to embrace and accommodate those among us with disabilities?), but becomes, as noted above, one for the individual woman to prevent (what will *she* do to avoid having a baby with a disability?).

Perhaps more troubling, however, prenatal testing implicitly assumes some norm of ability. Not only has testing clearly shaped attitudes toward Down syndrome, making it a privileged reason for abortion, but it gives social endorsement—if not active encouragement—to the abortion of a fetus on the basis of its potential ability.

Women have abortions for many reasons. No matter what one's commitment to women's reproductive freedom may be, however, some abortions seem more troubling than others. In this more problematic group are abortions that occur because society has created implicit expectations about the kinds of babies women should have. In so doing, society fails to provide women with what they require to be able to continue a wanted pregnancy to term, whether or not a disability has been identified. Unfortunately, prenatal testing contributes to this failure.

4. Prenatal testing further shapes the experience of abortion in ways beyond the models on which we usually rely to guarantee women's privacy and control. As suggested earlier, prenatal testing may not only reduce a woman's liberty to refuse an abortion, but it allows geneticists and their obstetrician colleagues to impose a "choice" for abortion covertly, if not overtly, when they decide which fetuses are healthy, what defines healthy, and who should be born. They do this merely by

offering tests for certain conditions and not others, as well as by what they tell parents about such conditions. (For a summary of these "twice-told" tales see Lippman & Wilfond, 1992.) That the birth of certain babies should be avoided is announced merely by making testing available. And as specialists in prenatal screening programs determine, more and more, whether a condition will be marginalized, an object of treatment, or grounds for abortion, the more power they gain over decisions to continue or terminate pregnancies—power that pregnant women themselves may not always have.

Prenatal testing shapes control over abortion, too, by legitimizing a role for insurance companies and governments in what should be an intensely personal matter for the individual woman. Whoever funds genetic testing programs or covers the cost of treatment for conditions diagnosable in utero may claim a say in determining which tests are carried out and what action the results must entail (Billings, 1990). Recent reports of the plan of a health maintenance organization in the United States to withdraw medical coverage if a child with cystic fibrosis was born whose birth could have been avoided by a "choice" to abort the pregnancy after the prenatal diagnosis was made (Billings et al., 1992) give substance to concerns about the power of testing to shape control of abortion.

However dramatic, such gross abuses should not distract us from the seemingly straightforward and everyday policies for testing programs that also reshape abortion choices. For example, women's decisions about pregnancy termination for the same chromosome abnormality are influenced by whether or not fetal anomalies are visualized on ultrasound (Drugan, Greb, Johnson, & Krivchenia, 1990). They are influenced too by the person who announces that an abnormality has been found, with rates of abortion reported as higher when the information is related by obstetricians than by geneticists (Holmes-Siedle, Ryynanen, & Lindenbaum, 1987). Even replacing amniocentesis by the earlier CVS reshapes control because geneticists generally view first trimester terminations as less problematic than the possibility of a second trimester termination and, thereby, a less legitimate reason to refuse prenatal testing.

No policy may have yet been formulated explicitly to reshape control over abortion, but shifts in control are embedded in the very process of testing (only some conditions are tested for, some person must provide counseling, some method must be used), and it is insufficient merely to consider the change in the locus of control as a "side effect" subject to regulation or ethical review. We can draft and enforce regulations that establish who shall do counseling, when and whether ultrasound scans will be shown, and so on, to avoid misuse, but every use will have some effect on abortion. And these effects will reflect the values of those with power and position to establish the policies.

5. Prenatal testing reshapes our perspective on a woman's life cycle. This stems from the subtle entanglement between prenatal diagnosis and another long-standing problematic issue for women—aging (Martin, 1987)—and from the ways in which development of testing around maternal age 35 has reflected and reinforced existing attitudes toward women and their adequacy. At the least, the availability of prenatal diagnosis and professionally imposed age limits on access to testing have created the social category of "the older woman" (Nelkin & Tancredi, 1989). More troublesome, however, is how testing is portrayed as a tool for the already negatively stereotyped woman in her middle years who wants or needs to circumvent features of aging. With this tool, the increasing probability of chromosomal nondisjunction associated with increases in a woman's age can be managed, just as cosmetic surgery and estrogen replacement regimens can manage her other bodily changes associated with getting older. The biological "failure" causing Down syndrome can be controlled and older women need not be "less fit" (Hubbard & Henifin, 1985) for childbearing, just as wrinkles of the skin or hot flashes that also make her "less fit" can be controlled. Against this background, the enthusiasm of medical researchers who have recently begun to create pregnancies in women well beyond menopause using eggs from younger women should certainly trouble us (Sauer, Paulson, & Lobo, 1990).

Prenatal testing for women 35 and older may not be as transparently age-ist as the use of donated or purchased ova to create a pregnancy in a postmenopausal woman, but it also reshapes the "older woman" by its reliance on chronological age or its equivalent as a principal criterion for fetal diagnosis. It implies that this sole feature is all that matters about a woman and conveys the message that after some arbitrary age she is a failure.

Given how prenatal genetic testing involves these various transformations—of pregnancy, of the fetus, of disability, of abortion as a choice, and of age—and the adaptions it demands of women, it becomes appropriate to see it as a lifestyle. Moreover, it is a lifestyle that takes for granted a very limited, class-biased, norm. How else would finding every fetus with Down syndrome become so important that universal triple screening is entering recommended medical practice while guaranteeing sufficient income and nutrition to all pregnant women to decrease their probability of having a premature or growth-retarded baby is not. The lifestyle of prenatal testing seems fashioned from a middle-class pattern that highlights the problems biomedical professionals themselves may experience. Women in this group are far more likely to have pregnancies when they are in their mid-30s and older than are poorer women, but they are much less likely to give birth to babies with growth problems.

Making Mothers Matter

When amniocentesis was introduced, abortion subsequent to the diagnosis of a fetal abnormality was presented as a temporary necessity until treatment for the detected condition could be devised. Advocates assumed that this would soon be forthcoming. With time, however, the gap between characterization and treatment of disease has widened. New information from efforts at gene mapping will certainly increase the ability to detect, diagnose, and screen, but not necessarily to treat. In fact, in the current sociopolitical climate of North America, where individual responsibility to prevent health problems takes precedence over social responsibility to support policies that promote the general well-being of all, developing remedies is probably far less likely than developing ways to prevent the birth of those who may have such problems.

The human gene map currently under construction will identify variations in DNA patterns. Genes alleged to cause specific disease, as well as those associated only with increased susceptibility to some disorder, will be found. All the variations that will be mapped could potentially become targets of prenatal testing. Which physical, mental, and aesthetic characteristics of our children do we want to select? Why? Do we want others to do this selection for us, as necessarily occurs when choices and needs are constructed by them?

Prenatal screening and testing are evolving in a climate that favors a genetic approach to personal and public health, an approach that is fundamentally expensive, individualized, and eugenic (Lippman, 1991, 1992a, 1992b). Giving that approach priority diminishes incentives to challenge the existing system that handicaps those with disabilities and makes it next to impossible for a woman to refuse an offer of testing or to choose to give birth to a child after in utero testing has indicated it may develop some medical problem. Recently, a genetic variation said to be associated with increased susceptibility to lead poisoning was described in the literature, with the authors implying this might be a useful objective of a screening program (Wetmur, Kaya, Plewinska, & Desnick, 1991). Do we really want to screen for genes rather than clean out lead to prevent the avoidable damage known to affect the millions of children unnecessarily exposed annually to this toxic agent (Lippman, 1992a)?

Although it is more than 20 years since the first fetal diagnosis of Down syndrome by amniocentesis, we still do not know the full impact of prenatal testing on women's total health, power, or social standing (Lippman, 1992c). For this reason alone, defining a place for prenatal screening and testing in our lives and in our health systems is not easy. Unfortunately, nor have we really grappled with the economic and eugenic forces propelling testing activities.

It would be naive to believe we can—or even would want to—dis-invent the technologies (though we might want to isolate rather than institutionalize them), but it might be an informative exercise to ask some fresh questions about how we might live without further extensions in the use of prenatal testing instead of examining only how we might implement them. Why not consider alternatives to geneticization before remediation (fixing it up) or regulation (keeping it ethical and legal) become our only demands?

Seeking such alternatives may be facilitated if we recall that variations in the distribution of wealth and power have far greater impact on the distribution of health than do variations in the distribution of genes. And both are inherited within families. Why do we construe childhood poverty as a "problem too big for ordinary mortals to tackle" (Heagarty, 1991), but consider mapping and sequencing all of the 50,000 to 100,000 human genes we have no big deal? Is children's development disrupted more by genetic loci than by ghetto lead? Do guns or genes alone cause more premature deaths in North America (cf. Novello, 1991)?

Health problems all have multiple causes, and to prevent ill health we must eliminate *some* cause—but it appears that *any* cause will do (Hesslow, 1984). We have social and medical options for dealing with genetic or any other disorders. Why do we segregate, for high priority, genetic services and programs to prevent the birth of those with potential for developing health problems?

Medical technology, prenatal genetic testing included, is especially seductive with its stories of human triumph. But unfortunately, the triumph for the individual who learns that her fetus does not have Down syndrome or some other detectable condition may not be a triumph for the collectives to which she and we all belong. We must never lose our compassion for an individual's situation, including her desire for reassurance, but we must also never forget that addressing often elastic private needs—needs that geneticists and obstetricians help to create—may dislocate provisions required for our collective health or solidify existing inequities in women's positions. And we might seriously consider that individual rights only have meaning within the relationships and collectivities of our lives.

Unfortunately, in considering issues of health and disease, some disjunction between individual wishes and societal needs will persist. The disjunction is being reinforced by genetic stories that more and more constrain notions of health and normality; that promote reliance on biomedical technology as a replacement for social and environmental change; and that privatize and individualize health problems. The disjunction is being played out in sterile debates too quickly (and falsely) polarized between pros and cons that trivialize the possible advantages and disadvantages of prenatal testing in response to women's valid health concerns. These debates incorrectly decontextualize testing, sever its essential relatedness to time and place, ignore the imbalances in power between the providers and users, and isolate it from the broader health and social policy agenda of which it is a part. The issue is not between experts promoting technology and Luddites trying to retard science. It is not between women who "want" prenatal diagnosis and women who don't want them to have it. It is not a dispute between advocates of prenatal diagnosis who are seen as defending women's already fragile rights to abortion and critics who are said to be fueling right-to-life supporters seeking to impose limits on women (and their choices).

Feminists concerned with how prenatal testing technology creates a coercive lifestyle for women and how the technology may be used to manipulate them are not "fetalists" (Raymond, 1987)—or fatalists. Recognizing the power imbalances between the providers and the users of testing, they are concerned about potential violence to women from the use of technology. They are seeking not to limit women's options but to ensure and expand them by exposing the structures that now constrain women's choices. To these critics—and I am among them—choice in prenatal testing means that it can be rejected by a woman without someone questioning her motives. It means that a woman could, if she wished, continue her pregnancy after a fetal diagnosis is made because we have guaranteed her help to support a child with a disability. And it means that personal actions are completely severed from public agendas so that a decrease in uptake rates from current levels might be seen to measure the effectiveness, not the failure, of prenatal screening (cf. Clarke, in press).

Prenatal testing is developed and applied with inherent expectations of how, when, and why it will be used that are tied to attitudes about women and about disability. It is currently expanding in a society that is deeply fractured along lines of gender, race, class, and ability. Its promotion and application can only reflect and, in turn, reinforce those divisions.

We need urgently, therefore, to question that technology not because of nostalgia for some seemingly simpler past, but because we recognize how political systems, cultural beliefs, and complex patterns of human relationships overlap, alter, and are altered by the application of screening. We need to question its power over us and its ways of controlling how we live without confusing the modern with the good, the newer with the better, or science with the objective, so as to grapple effectively with the extensive social modeling that testing tools allow.

Consequently, it is imperative that we continue to read the stories being told about prenatal genetic testing with a critical eye, situate them in time and place, question their assumptions, and demystify their language and metaphors. A healthy child is a matter of concern for all of us, mothers or not. But so is the world in which these children will live.

Women's desire for children without disability warrants complete public and private support. The question is how to provide support for women in a way that does no harm, that does not measure its effectiveness by the short-term profit from money saved when the lives of those with present or future disabilities are prevented, that does not view the birth of a child with a disability as a technological failure. Does support for expanded fetal screening programs improve how we welcome those with all kinds of abilities to our communities? Does the allocation of resources to genetic services correct gendered inequities and injustices in the health care system that endanger women's health? Is placing fetal screening in the routine prenatal care package part of the solution or part of the problem? Is its use liberating or oppressive or both—and for whom? Because we have a responsibility to mothers today as well as to the generations of those who present and future genetic testing programs will, or will not, allow to be born, and because the values and beliefs we transmit by engaging in the practice of prenatal genetic testing and selection will influence the possibilities for the next generation no less than will transmitted genes, we must not just ask but vigorously search for responses to these questions now.

ACKNOWLEDGMENTS

The contents of this chapter summarize, update, and expand upon material presented in Lippman 1992a and 1992b. The research on which this is based has been supported by the Social Sciences and Humanities Research Council of Canada.

My deepest thanks to Elizabeth Thomson and Karen Rothenberg for inviting me to participate in the National Institutes of Health conference they organized. This provided an especially rich and stimulating opportunity to meet, work with, befriend, and learn from a remarkable group of women. The friendships and collaborations initiated at this conference continue to nurture me and my ideas and have already helped me rethink many of the issues touched on in this chapter which is an updated version of previously published material. Thanks, too, to Vanessa Hill for enduring multiple revisions of the same material, organizing me as much as it.

NOTES

1. The use of prenatal genetic testing for the purposes of sex selection comes immediately to mind as perhaps the most blatant example.
2. For example, one factor in choosing age 35 in Canada was apparently the need to ensure that some smaller genetic centers would have a sufficient number of candidates to achieve the procedure rate required for a practitioner to meet professional standards. If a higher age were the cutoff, too few women would be tested to fulfill the standard minimum (Wyatt, personal communication, 1992).
3. Actually, only the number of things *called* genetic is increasing, not the number of genetic diseases themselves. This increase in "perceived" genetic disorders serves to legitimize offers of genetic help.

BIBLIOGRAPHY

ASCH, A. (1988). Reproductive technology and disability. In S. Cohen & N. Taub (Eds.), *Reproductive laws for the 1990s* (pp.59–101). Clifton, NJ: Humana Press.

BEESON, D. (1984). Technological rhythms in pregnancy. In T. Duster & K. Garrett (Eds.), *Cultural perspectives on biological knowledge* (pp. 145–181). Norwood, NJ: Ablex.

BILLINGS, P. (1990). Genetic discrimination: An ongoing survey. *Gene-WATCH, 6*(4/5), 7–15.

BILLINGS, P., Kohn, M. A., de Cuevas, M., Beckwith, J., Alper, J. S., & Natowicz, M. R. (1992). Genetic discrimination as a consequence of genetic screening. *American Journal of Human Genetics, 50,* 476–482.

CLARKE, A. (in press). Response to "What counts as success in genetics counselling?" In *Ethical aspects of genetic counselling*. London: Routledge.

DRUGAN, A., Greb, A., Johnson, M. P., & Krivchenia, E. L. (1990). Determinants of parental decisions to abort for chromosome abnormalities. *Prenatal Diagnosis, 10*(8), 483–490.

DUMEZ, Y. (1989). L'amniocentèse: Un examen courant. *Science & Vie, 169*, 56–57.

EWING, C. (1990). Australian perspectives on embryo experimentation: An update. *Issues in Reproductive Genetic Engineering, 3*(2), 119–123.

FARRANT, W. (1985). Who's for amniocentesis? The politics of prenatal screening. In H. Homans (Ed.), *The sexual politics of reproduction* (pp. 96–122). Aldershot, England: Gower.

GREEN, J., Statham, H., & Snowdon, C. (1992). Screening for fetal abnormalities: Attitudes and experiences. In T. Chard & M. P. M. Richards (Eds.), *Obstetrics in the 1990s: Current controversies* (pp. 65–89). London: MacKeith Press.

HEAGARTY, M. (1991). America's lost children: Whose responsibility? *Journal of Pediatrics, 118*, 8.

HILL, E. C. (1986). Your morality or mine? An inquiry into the ethics of human reproduction. *American Journal of Obstetrics and Gynecology, 154*, 1173–1180.

HOLMES-SIEDLE, M., Ryynanen, M., & Lindenbaum, R. H. (1987). Parental decisions regarding termination of pregnancy affecting prenatal detection of sex chromosome abnormality. *Prenatal Diagnosis, 7*, 239–244.

HUBBARD, R. (1984). Personal courage is not enough: Some hazards of childbearing in the 1980s. In R. Arditti, R. D. Klein, & S. Minden (Eds.), *Test-tube women* (pp. 331–355). London: Pandora.

HUBBARD, R., & Henifin, M. S. (1985). Genetic screening of prospective parents and of workers: Some scientific and social issues. *International Journal of Health Services, 15*(2), 231–251.

KUITERT, H. M. (1988). Using genetic data: A moral assessment of the direct social consequences. In H. Rigter, J. C. F. Bletz, A. Krijnen, B. Wijnberg, & H. D. Banta (Eds.), *The social consequences of genetic testing* (p. 31) [Proceedings of a Conference, Leidschendam]. The Hague: Netherlands Scientific Council for Government Policy.

LIPPMAN, A. (1986). Access to prenatal screening services: Who decides? *Canadian Journal of Women and Law, 1*, 434–445.

LIPPMAN, A. (1989). Prenatal diagnosis: Reproductive choice? Reproductive control? In C. Overall (Ed.), *The future of human reproduction* (pp. 182–194). Toronto: Women's Press.

LIPPMAN, A. (1991). Prenatal genetic testing and screening: Constructing needs and reinforcing inequities. *American Journal of Law and Medicine, 17*(1 & 2), 15–50.

LIPPMAN, A. (1992a). Led (astray) by genetic maps: The cartography of the human genome and health care. *Social Science Medicine, 35*(12), 1469–1476.

LIPPMAN, A. (1992b). Mother matters: A fresh look at prenatal genetic testing. *Issues in Reproductive Genetic Engineering, 5*(2), 141–154.

LIPPMAN, A. (1992c). Prenatal diagnosis: Can what counts be counted? *Women & Health, 18*(2), 1–8.

LIPPMAN-HAND, A., & Fraser, F. C. (1979a). Genetic counseling: The post-counseling period. I. Parents' perceptions of uncertainty. *American Journal of Medical Genetics, 4*, 51–71.

LIPPMAN-HAND, A., & Fraser, F. C. (1979b). Genetic counseling: The postcounseling period. II. Making reproductive choices. *American Journal of Medical Genetics, 4*, 73–87.

LIPPMAN, A., Messing, K., & Mayer, F. (1990). Commentary: Is genome mapping the way to improve Canadians' health? *Canadian Journal of Public Health, 81*, 397–398.

LIPPMAN, A., & Wilfond, B. S. (1992). "Twice-told tales": Stories about genetic disorders. *American Journal of Human Genetics, 51*, 936–937.

MARTIN, E. (1987). *The woman in the body: A cultural analysis of reproduction.* Boston: Beacon Press.

MOATTI, J. P., Lanoë, J.-L., LeGalès, C., Gardent, H., Julian, C., & Aymé, S. (1989, September). Economic assessment of prenatal diagnosis in France. Paper presented at Joint Meeting of European Health Economic Societies, Barcelona, Spain.

MYERS, G. (1990). The double helix as icon. *Science as Culture, 9*, 49–72.

NELKIN, D., & Tancredi, L. (1989). *Dangerous diagnostics: The social power of biological information.* New York: Basic Books.

NOVELLO, A. C. (1991). Violence is a greater killer of children than disease. *Public Health Reports, 106*, 231.

PRESS, N. A., & Browner, C. H. (1993). Collective fictions: Similarities in the reasons for accepting MSAFP screening among women of diverse ethnic and social class backgrounds. *Fetal Diagnosis Therapy, 8* (Supp. 1), 97–106.

QUÉNIART, A. (1988). Le corps paradoxal. In *Regards de femmes sur le maternité.* Montréal: Editions St. Martin.

RAPP, R. (1988). The power of "positive" diagnosis: Medical and maternal discourses on amniocentesis. In K. L. Michaelson (Ed.), *Childbirth in America: Anthropological perspectives* (pp. 103–116). Hadley, MA: Bergin & Garvey.

RAYMOND, J. (1987). Fetalists and feminists: They are not the same. In P. Spallone & D. L. Steinberg (Eds.), *Made to order* (pp. 58–66). New York: Pergamon Press.

RETSINAS, J. (1991). The impact of prenatal testing upon attitudes toward disabled infants. *Research in Social Health Care, 9*, 75–102.

ROBERTSON, J. A. (1983). Procreative liberty and the control of conception, pregnancy and childbirth. *Virginia Law Review, 69*, 405–464.

ROSENBERG, C. E. (1992). Introduction. In C. E. Rosenberg & J. Golden (Eds.), *Framing disease: Studies in cultural history*. New Brunswick, NJ: Rutgers University Press.

ROTHMAN, B. K (1986). *The tentative pregnancy: Prenatal diagnosis and the future of motherhood*. New York: Viking.

ROTHMAN, B. K. (1989). *Recreating motherhood: Ideology and technology in a patriarchal society*. New York: Norton.

ROWLAND, R. (1984). Reproductive technologies: The final solution to the woman question. In R. Arditti, R. D. Klein, & S. Minden (Eds.), *Test-tube women* (pp. 356–369). London: Pandora.

ROYAL College of Physicians of London. (1989). *Prenatal diagnosis and genetic screening: Community and service implications*. London: Royal College of Physicians.

SAUER, M. V., Paulson, R. J., & Lobo, R. A. (1990). A preliminary report on oocyte donation extending reproductive potential to women over 40. *New England Journal of Medicine, 323*(17), 1157–1160.

SHAPIRO, R. (1990). The human blueprint. [Lecture, Science College Public Lecture Series, 29 November, 1990]. Concordia Univ., Montreal.

SHAW, M. (1980). The potential plaintiff: Preconceptional and prenatal torts. In A. Milunsky & G. J. Annas (Eds.), *Genetics and the law II*. New York: Plenum.

VEKEMANS, M., & Lippman, A. (1984). Eligibility criteria for amniocentesis. *American Journal of Medical Genetics, 17*, 531–533, 539.

WETMUR, J. G., Kaya, A. H., Plewinska, M., & Desnick, R. J. (1991). Molecular characterization of the human δ-aminolevulinate dehydratase 2 (ALAD²) allele: Implications for molecular screening of individuals for genetic susceptibility to lead poisoning. *American Journal of Human Genetics, 49*, 757–763.

WRIGHT, P. W. G., & Treacher, A. (Eds.). (1982). *The problem of medical knowledge*. Edinburgh: University of Edinburgh Press.

2 Women's Roles in the History of Amniocentesis and Chorionic Villi Sampling

RUTH SCHWARTZ COWAN

The history of the modern forms of prenatal diagnosis is not a very long story, as historical narratives go, but it is longer than most people think; it starts in about 1950, 40 years ago. In addition it is a complex story because prenatal diagnosis is a complex technology. Indeed, prenatal diagnosis should properly be thought of as a sociotechnological system composed of several subsidiary parts: the medical delivery services that convince women to become patients; the means of obtaining fetal tissue from those patients; biochemical assays of the tissue; the culturing and karyotyping of fetal cells; molecular analysis of fetal DNA; ultrasound examination and guidance; and abortion. Each part of the system has its own scientific history and its own inseparable social history and, to make matters even more complicated, those separate histories have transpired in many different countries, under many different social, economic, and scientific conditions.[1]

This chapter focuses only on a small portion of that complex of histories, that portion which is concerned with the means of obtaining fetal tissue for diagnosis. I have chosen to examine the histories of amniocentesis and chorionic villi sampling (CVS)—as well as what remains the only available therapy for a positive diagnosis, abortion—because doing so allows me to look at particular aspects of women's roles in the history of prenatal diagnosis and to make certain suggestions about what policy directions seem most likely to achieve the necessary goals in the United States.

Historians and other students of technology make a useful distinction when they discuss technological change—that between the developmental phases and the diffusion phases of a technology. Although it is not always an easy distinction to make, roughly speaking, when a technology is in development it is changing rapidly and being applied narrowly, under various kinds of testing conditions. When it is in diffusion, as the word suggests, it is spreading; its form is more or less fixed—or changing only slowly—and it is coming into routine use, becoming embedded in, we might say, a social matrix.

Amniocentesis is now in diffusion and has been since the late 1970s; chorionic villi sampling, on the other hand, has only recently started to diffuse and may arguably (at the date of publication) still be in the last stages of development. The distinction between development and diffusion is important to keep in mind because when a technology shifts from development to diffusion the cast of important social actors shifts with it; those who have the power to make changes in development are not those who have the power to make changes in diffusion.

The two most common means today for obtaining fetal tissue are amniocentesis and chorionic villi sampling. Amniocentesis came first. The amniotic tap itself, the low-tech part of the procedure, had become a routine part of obstetric practice by at least the mid-1950s, in part because it was used in the third trimester, sometimes to relieve patients with hydramnios, and sometimes to permit biochemical testing of the incompatibility between Rh-negative mothers and their fetuses (Fuchs & Cederqvist, 1970).

In 1949 Murray L. Barr and his colleagues discovered that the cells of female and male mammals could be distinguished from each other by the presence or absence, not of sex chromosomes (which in those years were very difficult to see under the microscope), but of another, very small, cellular body, which has since been named after him—the Barr body, or sex chromatin. Females seemed to have it and males didn't, so it could be used to ascertain sex where that was anatomically or visually unclear; sex chromatin is visible under the microscope even when cells are not in active division. By 1953 Barr and his coworkers had discovered that sex chromatin was characteristic in humans as well as in cats and mice (Moore, Graham, & Barr, 1953).

In the 1950s a small group of medical specialists, medical geneticists, were interested in ascertaining sex when it was neither anatomically nor visually obvious in order to discover the sex of fetuses being carried by women with family histories of sex-linked diseases such as hemophilia. Such patients were referred to medical geneticists for consultations about whether to have children, whether it was wise to marry a specific person, or whether a specific pregnancy should be carried to term. Medical geneticists, unfortunately, had no diagnostic techniques to offer except the construction and analysis of a sometimes faulty family medical history. In most cases the diagnoses were little more than probability statements: "The chances are 50–50 that your child will be afflicted," or, "The chances are very slim that your partner will carry the same recessive gene that you do." Not surprisingly, both patients and specialists found this to be a tragically frustrating enterprise (Hammons, 1959). Barr's discovery, however, held the promise of relieving a small portion of this frustration. If a woman had been identified as a carrier of the gene and if the sex of her fetus could be determined in utero, the geneticist could predict with much greater certainty (albeit not with complete certainty) whether the child, when born, would have hemophilia (Macintyre, 1973).

Four different groups of researchers are credited with the discovery in 1955 that the sex of human fetuses could be predicted through analysis of fetal cells in amniotic fluid: one each in New York, Minneapolis, Copenhagen, and Haifa (Shettles, 1956; Makowski, 1956; Fuchs & Riis, 1956; Serr, Sachs, & Danon, 1955). A short while later the Copenhagen group became the first to report that they had performed an abortion in order to prevent the birth of a fetus, diagnosed as being male, whose mother was a carrier of hemophilia (Riis & Fuchs, 1960). Prenatal diagnosis through amniocentesis was, if you will excuse the pun, born; the year was 1960.

Amniocentesis remained in its developmental stages for another 15 years, partly because it took several years for techniques to be developed for the diagnosis of fetal conditions other than sex, partly because it took that long for the safety of the procedure to be ascertained, and partly because Scandinavia was the only place, for much of that time, in which so-called eugenic therapeutic abortions could be legally performed and obtained (Callahan, 1970). We can assume, although documentation is difficult to produce, that outside of Scandinavia prenatal diagnosis for sex was performed on a very limited number of pregnant women—those who had been referred to specialists because of a family history of a known sex-linked hereditary disease—and only in a few medical research centers whose staff were willing to "look the other way" when a D&C was ordered. We can also assume (although, again, documentation is difficult to produce), that most of those women believed that the D&Cs were in their best interests; they knew what it was like to have hemophilia, for example, or to be the parent of a child with hemophilia, and they were willing to go to considerable trouble to have the operation performed (Macintyre, 1973).

In 1959 a French cytogeneticist, Jerome LeJeune, discovered that one common form of Down syndrome was caused by trisomy of the 21st chromosome, and at that point several medical geneticists realized that there was a wider potential for amniocentesis if some way could be found to culture fetal cells successfully; because the cells in amniotic fluid are neither numerous nor in active division, mitotic figures were few and far between, making karyotyping exceedingly difficult (LeJeune, Gauthier, & Turpin, 1959a, 1959b). The culturing problem was solved, seven years later, in 1966 (Steele & Breg, 1966). The first abortions after midtrimester amniocentesis and karyotyping were reported very shortly thereafter, in 1968, and the cooperative registry, intended to ascertain the safety of the procedure was begun in the United States in 1971 (Nadler, 1968; Valenti, Schutta, & Kehaty, 1968). When the results of those trials were announced in the fall of 1975, and finally published in the winter of 1976, the developmental stage of amniocentesis can be said to have been drawing to a close (NICHD, 1976).

The equipment needed for the amniotic tap was not particularly expensive and the skills were relatively easy to learn. Many of the larger hospitals and clinics had already purchased devices for obstetric ultrasound, which could be used to ascertain the position of the fetus. Ever larger populations of potential patients could be anticipated, just over the horizon, since the presenting symptom "advanced maternal age" is more widely distributed in the population than the presenting symptom of having a family history of a sex-linked hereditary disease. Therapeutic eugenic abortion, along with other forms of abortion, had, in the intervening years, become legal in the United States, Canada, and Britain, in addition to Scandinavia. Diffusion was about to begin.

In the United States the events which, possibly more than any other, were responsible for kicking amniocentesis out of development and into diffusion, were the settlement in 1978 and 1979 of several lawsuits in which parents of children with a disability successfully sued for malpractice when an obstetrician had failed to refer a patient over the age of 35 for amniocentesis (Rogers, 1982). In one of the first of those cases, Dolores Becker, who was 37 years old when she became pregnant, was awarded her child's medical costs for life (Becker, 1978). The American College of Obstetricians and Gynecologists and the American Academy of Pediatrics subsequently advised their members that, henceforth, they had better offer prenatal diagnostic services or referrals for prenatal diagnosis to their patients, or risk the same kind of suit (American Academy, 1983).

Three analytic points about the role of women in the history of amniocentesis can be made at this juncture in the story. First, the initial stages of development were determined, in part, by the ways in which research physicians interpreted the behavior of their female patients. In the period between 1955 and 1975 some women voluntarily presented themselves as eager recipients of counseling from medical geneticists. Some of these women willingly submitted to the experimental trials of amniocentesis, and some sought eugenic therapeutic abortions when there was hardly any hope of finding one. None of those women sued their physicians (or even complained publicly) for offering advice that was not requested, or for performing a diagnostic procedure that was not wanted; if there were women who felt that their interests or their rights had been ignored or diminished during this early period, they have left no trace of their sentiments in the public record. Amniocentesis was designed by research physicians who believed, with considerable justification, that they were acting in the best interests of their patients, patients who were, let us remember, at very high risk for becoming the parents of afflicted children. The physicians perceived, also with considerable justification, that their patients were grateful for the services—however rudimentary—that were being offered.

Second, amniocentesis would not have passed out of the developmental stage into the diffusion stage unless the abortion laws in the United States, Canada, and Britain had been reformed. Since many women played various active roles in working for the reformation of those laws, we must conclude that through their organized activity, as well as through their individual efforts, some women acted so as to make prenatal diagnosis possible, whether they were conscious of the effects of their actions or not.

Third, the women who, like Dolores Becker, sued for wrongful birth acted (whether they realized it or not) in such a way as to ensure that prenatal diagnostic services would become a routine part of obstetric care—at least in the United States, and at least in those parts of the medical system in which patients interact with private practitioners on a fee-for-service basis. Not all technologies that go through development also go through diffusion; indeed the vast majority of new technologies fail to make the transition. Even those that go into the diffusion stage sometimes fail there, either because they do not find, or fail to create, a niche in the market. That amniocentesis made the transition and made it successfully is at least partly due to the individual actions of women who, presumably acting in what they thought to be their own best interests, sued their obstetricians for malpractice.

Chorionic villi sampling has had, in some ways, a more torturous history than amniocentesis. The first efforts to biopsy the chorion were made by Jan Mohr and Niels Hahnemann in Copenhagen in the late 1960s (Mohr, 1968; Hahnemann, 1974). The instrument that they used (and designed) was 6 mm in diameter; it contained a fiber-optic device for direct visualization of the chorion (Mohr, 1968). Living and working in Copenhagen, Mohr was one of the few medical geneticists in the world at that time who had had considerable experience in diagnosing birth defects through amniocentesis and in referring patients for midtrimester abortions. In one of their early papers Mohr and Hahnemann stated their reasons for exploring a diagnostic technique that could be done in the first rather than second trimester: "On considerations regarding the mental and physical health of the mother, and also for legal reasons, it seems essential to establish such a diagnosis as early in pregnancy as possible" (Hahnemann & Mohr, 1968, p. 47). Mohr, in a subsequent interview, has explained what he meant more precisely. Women who desired therapeutic abortions after amniocentesis were, he believes, humiliated by the paperwork that was required in order to obtain permission for such an abortion from the panel of physicians that Danish law then required (Mohr, personal communication, May 1989, June 1992). Mohr and Hahnemann's trials were not successful; they had what they regarded as an unacceptably high miscarriage rate and considerable difficulty in culturing the cells. They abandoned their efforts in 1974 (Mohr, 1968). A year earlier a pair of Swedish researchers had reported more promising results using an instrument 5 mm in diameter, but there was no follow-up to their initial study (Kullander & Sandahl, 1973). In 1975 a team of Chinese researchers published an article in which they reported efforts they had made over a period of several years to diagnose the sex of fetuses, without cell culture, using an exceedingly simple instrument (no fiber optics, an essentially blind approach). They reported 100 attempts, out of which 82 produced vaginal smears and three resulted in spontaneous abortion; there were six incorrect diagnoses and 30 induced abortions, of which 29 were of females (Tietung, 1975).

With the exception of one unsuccessful effort to get chorionic cells by uterine lavage (Goldberg, Chen, Ahn, & Reidy, 1980), nothing else appeared in the literature on chorionic villi sampling (or biopsy, as it was then called) until a spate of articles late in 1982 and in the early months of 1983. One team, working under the aegis of the former Soviet Union's Ministry of Health, reported on 165 biopsies using an embryo-fetoscope 1.7 mm in diameter in which they had considerable success in obtaining tissue, in not causing pregnancy loss, in diagnosis of sex, and also in several biochemical diagnostic analyses (Kazy, Rosovsky, & Bakharev, 1982). Two British groups reported using real-time ultrasound and a more flexible and even narrower (1.5 mm) biopsy instrument in the diagnosis of the hemoglobinopathies, through molecular analysis (Williamson et al., 1981; Old et al., 1982). A third British group, using a somewhat different instrument, reported success in determining fetal sex through molecular analysis of DNA (Gosden, Mitchell, Gosden, Rodeck, & Morsman, 1982). Within months a French group was using yet another instrument to take samples and diagnose sickle-cell anemia, and an Italian group was beginning to perfect a technique for direct karyotyping of chorionic tissue, without the need to wait for culturing (Goossens et al., 1983; Simoni, Brambati, & Danesino, 1983). Under the auspices of the World Health Organization, a working group on first trimester fetal diagnosis met in April, 1984, in Geneva, and a full-scale international conference on the subject was held in Rapallo, Italy, six months later (WHO, 1984).

An enormous amount of developmental research work has been done on chorionic villi sampling in the intervening years. Some of this work has been devoted to perfecting an instrument that will be both relatively easy to manipulate and reasonably nonintrusive. Other work has been devoted to standardizing the techniques for karyotyping, molecular analysis, and biochemical assaying of chorionic tissue. Yet other work has been devoted to assessing the safety of the procedure—safety gauged in terms of pregnancy loss as well as in terms of maternal and child health.[2]

Yet it is possible to assert that, at least for the United States, chorionic villi sampling has, for the moment, been stalled in its developmental phase; many knowledgeable people question whether it will, or should, ever emerge into diffusion, especially in view of the recent claims that sampling increases the likelihood of birth defects (Firth et al., 1989). The reasons for this delay, despite what many claim to be very clear advantages of a first trimester diagnostic technique, seem multiple and varied. There is always a competitive advantage for the technology that gets to the marketplace first—and amniocentesis got there first. Since the techniques for chorionic biopsy are harder for practitioners to learn, this recency means that CVS was initially bound to be less safe than amniocentesis.

But something else is operating in the story of the delayed diffusion of chorionic villi sampling. "Social pressures in the United States," one participant observed, "were antagonistic to the development of new fetal diagnostic techniques" (Modell, 1986, p. 14). Between 1980 and the early months of 1993, clinical research on chorionic villi sampling was impeded by the various and sundry prohibitions against the use of federal funds for fetal research. Counterfactual history ("What would have happened if . . . ") is always a risky undertaking, but there are very good reasons to believe that had American research teams, and other research teams assisted with federal funding from the United States, been able to work as intensively on chorionic villi sampling as they had once worked on amniocentesis, it is possible—at least in the United States—that we might be much closer to diffusion of the technique than we are today. In an ironic way the politics of abortion in the 1970s helped to move amniocentesis out of development and into diffusion, while the anti-abortion politics of the 1980s worked to keep chorionic villi sampling from making the same transition.

Women have influenced the development of chorionic villi sampling in two of the same ways in which they influenced the development of amniocentesis: by their behavior as patients and by their participation in abortion reform movements, most notably those in France and Italy. The women who as patients stimulated (through their willingness to be patients, through their gratitude for the services provided, and through their return visits) the developmental work on chorionic villi sampling were, however, very different from the women who as patients first stimulated the development of amniocentesis. Many were neither white nor middle class: Pakistani women living in London; African women, many of them Muslims, living in France; Chinese women in Anshan; and Russian and Hungarian women. Yet something about their behavior, as perceived by the physicians whom they came to consult, convinced those physicians that first trimester prenatal diagnosis and first trimester abortion would ease their burdens as mothers. As Modell (1986) put

it, "Earlier diagnosis seemed particularly necessary because of
the social and religious attitudes of some ethnic groups at risk.
For instance, British Muslims originating from Pakistan are as
distressed as anyone else by having children suffering from thalassemia major, but most find midtrimester diagnosis and abortion unacceptable. *However they expressed a lively interest in the
possibility of first trimester diagnosis* [italics added]" (p. 14). In the
United States most of the women requesting prenatal diagnostic
services (and most of those who participated as patients in research trials) have been white women of above-average income
and educational levels, but the history of chorionic villi biopsy
teaches us that there are circumstances in which women who do
not fit in any of those categories have played a role in technological change.

Historians are, in general, uncomfortable making predictions
about the future, but I believe that it is possible to learn some
lessons from these stories about the history of prenatal diagnosis that can provide guidance about future policy options. First,
there is every reason to believe that women can affect the future
of prenatal diagnosis because they have, in the various ways I
have tried to specify, affected its past. Second, I believe the
chances of putting a brake on the progress of prenatal diagnosis—a brake that some feminist groups have recently advocated—are very slim, not just because medical genetics is now
a well established specialty, not just because various governments have, for various reasons, ulterior motives in promoting
prenatal diagnosis, but also because large groups of women, in
several different countries, of several different social classes,
very much want the services that medical geneticists can provide. Third, the only mechanism that I can see, on the basis of
my view of the past, for applying that brake will be to outlaw
abortion, a mechanism that—whatever its other faults may
be—very few activist women are going to be convinced to advocate. Fourth, those who believe that women's interests will
be best served by the diffusion of chorionic villi sampling and
by the development and diffusion of noninvasive diagnostic
techniques ought to pay attention to the fate of fetal research;
the ban that was recently overturned by one president's executive order may just as easily be reinstated by another's. Fifth,

and finally, those who believe that one desideratum for change is to extend prenatal diagnosis services to all sectors of the American population—especially to those who are poor or members of minority groups—need to think through, very carefully, not only the social and ethical pros and cons of such services, but also the pros and cons of malpractice suits as devices for ensuring the diffusion of medical technologies.

NOTES

1. There are no published histories of prenatal diagnosis that are comprehensive or that integrate the social, scientific, medical, and technical aspects of that history; the author is currently writing one. Parts of that history can be examined, however, in Cowan (1992), Cederqvist & Fuchs (1970), and Modell (1986).
2. For a review of the literature on the safety of chorionic villi sampling see Martins & Johnson (1993), Canadian Collaborative CVS-Amniocentesis Clinical Trial Group (1989), and MRC Working Party on the Evaluation of Chorionic Villus Sampling (1991).

BIBLIOGRAPHY

AMERICAN Academy of Pediatrics and American College of Obstetricians and Gynecologists. (1983). *Guidelines for perinatal care.*

BECKER v. Schwartz. (1978). 46 NY 2nd 401, 386 NE 2nd 807.

CALLAHAN, D. (1970). *Abortion: Law, choice, and morality.* New York: Macmillan.

CANADIAN Collaborative CVS-Amniocentesis Clinical Trial Group. (1989). Multicenter randomized clinical trial of chorionic villus sampling and amniocentesis. *Lancet, 331,* 11–13.

CEDERQVIST, L. L., & Fuchs, F. (1970). Antenatal sex determination: An historical review. *Clinical Obstetrics and Gynecology, 13,* 159–177.

COWAN, R. S. (1992). Genetic technology and reproductive choice: An ethics for autonomy. In D. J. Kevles & L. Hood (Eds.), *The code of codes: Scientific and social issues in the human genome project.* Cambridge, MA: Harvard University Press.

FIRTH, H. V., Boyd, P. A., Chamberlain, P., et al. (1989). Severe limb abnormalities after chorionic villus sampling at 56–66 days' gestation. *Lancet, 337,* 726.

FUCHS, F., & Cederqvist, L. (1970). Recent advances in antenatal diagnosis by amniotic fluid analysis. *Clinical Obstetrics and Gynecology, 13,* 178–201.

FUCHS, F., & Riis, P. (1956). Antenatal sex determination. *Nature, 177,* 330.

GOLDBERG, M. F., Chen, A., Ahn, Y. W., & Reidy, J. (1980). First trimester fetal chromosome diagnosis using endocervical lavage: A negative evaluation. *American Journal of Obstetrics and Gynecology, 138,* 436–440.

GOOSSENS, M., Dumez, Y., Kaplan, L., Lupker, M., Chabret, C., Henrion, R., & Rosa, J. (1983). Prenatal diagnosis of sickle-cell anemia in the first trimester of pregnancy. *New England Journal of Medicine, 309,* 831–833.

GOSDEN, J. R., Mitchell, A. R., Gosden, C. M., Rodeck, C. H., & Morsman, J. M. (1982). Direct vision chorion biopsy and chromosome specific DNA probes for determination of fetal sex in first trimester prenatal diagnosis. *Lancet, 2,* 1416–1419.

HAHNEMANN, N. (1974). Early prenatal diagnosis: A study of biopsy techniques and cell culturing from extraembryonic membranes. *Clinical Genetics, 6,* 294–306.

HAHNEMANN, N., & Mohr, J. (1969). Antenatal foetal diagnosis in genetic disease. *Bulletin of European Social and Human Genetics, 3,* 47.

HAMMONS, H. G. (Ed.). (1959). *Heredity counseling.* New York: Harper.

KAZY, Z., Rosovsky, I. S., & Bakharev, V. A. (1982). Chorion biopsy in early pregnancy: A method of early prenatal diagnosis for inherited disorders. *Prenatal Diagnosis, 2,* 39–45.

KULLANDER, S., & Sandahl, B. (1973). Fetal chromosomal analysis after transcervical placental biopsies during early pregnancy. *Acta Obstetrica et Gynecologica Scandinavia, 52,* 355–359.

LEJEUNE, J., Gauthier, M., & Turpin, R. (1959a). Les chromosomes humains en culture de tissus. *Comptes Rendus de l'Academie des Sciences, 248,* 602–603.

LEJEUNE, J., Gauthier, M., & Turpin, R. (1959b). Etudes des chromosomes somatiques de neuf enfants mongoliens. *Comptes Rendus de l'Academie des Sciences, 248,* 1721–1722.

MACINTYRE, M. N. (1973). Genetic risk, prenatal diagnosis and selective abortion. In D. F. Walbert & D. Butler (Eds.), *Abortion, society and the law* (pp. 234–252). Cleveland, OH: Case Western Reserve University Press.

MAKOWSKI, E. L., Prem, K. A., & Kaiser, I. H. (1956). Detection of sex of fetuses by the incidence of sex chromatin body in nuclei of cells in amniotic fluid. *Science, 123,* 542.

MARTINS, M., & Johnson, A. (1993). Does chorionic villus sampling cause limb defects? *Genetics and Teratology, 2*(1), 1–3.

MODELL, B. (1986). Fetal diagnosis in the first trimester: Introduction and historical perspective. In B. Brambati (Ed.), *Chorionic villus sampling: Fetal diagnosis of genetic disease in the first trimester* (pp. 1–16). New York: Dekker.

MOHR, J. (1968). Foetal genetic diagnosis: Development of techniques for early sampling of foetal cells. *Acta Pathologica et Microbiologica Scandinavia, 73*, 73–77.

MOORE, K. L., Graham, M., & Barr, M. L. (1953). The detection of chromosomal sex in hermaphrodites from a skin biopsy. *Surgical Gynecology and Obstetrics, 96*, 641–648.

MRC Working Party on the Evaluation of Chorionic Villus Sampling. (1991). Medical research council European trial of chorionic villus sampling. *Lancet, 337*, 1491.

NADLER, H. L. (1968). Antenatal detection of hereditary disorders. *Pediatrics, 42*, 912.

NICHD National Registry for Amniocentesis Study Group. (1976). Midtrimester amniocentesis for prenatal diagnosis: Safety and accuracy. *Journal of the American Medical Association, 236*, 1471–1476.

OLD, J. M., Ward, R. H. T., Karagozlu, F., Petrou, M., Modell, B., & Weatherall, D. J. (1982). First trimester fetal diagnosis for haemoglobinopathies: Three cases. *Lancet, 2*, 1414–1416.

RIIS, P., & Fuchs, F. (1960). Antenatal determination of foetal sex in prevention of hereditary diseases. *Lancet, 2*, 180.

ROGERS, T. D. (1982). Wrongful life and wrongful birth: Medical malpractice in genetic counselling and prenatal testing. *Science Law Review, 33*, 713.

SERR, D. M., Sachs, L., & Danon, M. (1955). Diagnosis of sex before birth using cells from the amniotic fluid. *Bulletin of the Research Council of Israel, 5B*, 137.

SHETTLES, L. B. (1956). Nuclear morphology of cells in human amniotic fluid in relation to sex of infant. *American Journal of Obstetrics and Gynecology, 71*, 834.

SIMONI, G., Brambati, B., & Danesino, C. (1983). Efficient direct chromosome analysis and enzyme determination from chorionic villi samples in the first trimester of pregnancy. *Human Genetics, 63*, 349–357.

STEELE, M. W., & Breg, W. R. (1966). Chromosome analysis of human amniotic fluid cells. *Lancet, 1*, 383.

TIETUNG Hospital Department of Obstetrics and Gynecology. (1975). Fetal sex prediction by sex chromatin of chorionic villi cells during early pregnancy. *Chinese Medical Journal, 1*, 117–126.

VALENTI, C., Schutta, E. J., & Kehaty, T. (1968). Prenatal diagnosis of Down's syndrome. *Lancet, 2*, 220.

WHO Working Group. (1984). Fetal diagnosis of hereditary diseases. *Bulletin of the World Health Organization, 62*, 345–355.

WILLIAMSON, R., Eskdale, J., Coleman, D. V., Niazi, N., Loeffler, F. E., & Modell, B. (1981). Direct gene analysis of chorionic villi: A possible technique for first trimester antenatal diagnosis of haemoglobinpathies. *Lancet, 2*, 1125–1127.

3 Prenatal Screening and Diagnosis:

The Impact on Persons with Disabilities

DEBORAH KAPLAN

The disability rights movement has come of age in the 1990s with the passage of the Americans with Disabilities Act and with increased public attention to disability concerns. Persons with disabilities have made great advances in moving social policy away from two different models of thought on disability: the "charity" approach, which presumes that the best we can do is to provide welfare and charity toward primarily custodial services for persons with less social value, and the "medical" approach, which applies a medical framework toward social problems presented by disability and assumes that the best outcome is for a medical cure of the disability. A new approach, based on integrating persons with disabilities into society and accepting disability as a predictable aspect of life, has emerged during the past two decades.

Prenatal screening is inherently concerned with the existence, or avoidance, of disability in society and individuals. Are the social goals of those who have worked for the widespread use of prenatal screening consistent with those of the disability rights movement? As persons with disabilities have moved into significant policy-making positions throughout society, their views and experiences are becoming difficult to ignore.

The purpose of this chapter is to examine some of the policy implications of prenatal screening from a disability perspective. That perspective is based on the life experiences of persons with disabilities who have attained academic, scientific, and social roles that provide them with an opportunity to present a new way of looking at the value of living with a disability. This chapter also reviews some of the most commonly given reasons for prenatal screening and extracts potential research topics from an analysis of those reasons.

Why Do We Engage in Prenatal Testing?

The most frequently given reason for utilizing prenatal testing is that we are trying to prevent or ameliorate medical or disabling conditions that are genetically based. Once a genetic syndrome or condition is diagnosed in a fetus, there are three types of prevention that can be pursued:

1. Prevention of the birth through abortion. Although new testing procedures sometimes permit this to take place during the first trimester of pregnancy, many such abortions still occur during the second trimester.

2. Prevention or amelioration of the disability using methods such as treatment through dietary changes or supplements for the mother or infant; prenatal treatment of the fetus through pharmaceutical or surgical interventions; other forms of treatment or therapy for the infant that occur after prenatal diagnosis.

3. Prevention of family disruption through prenatal preparation by family members. This can entail obtaining information about the diagnosed condition and its consequences through reading or through talking to families who have children with similar disabilities or to adults who live with the disability themselves. It may also include such means as finding out about available public or private resources or forms of assistance, purchasing equipment, or making home modifications.

From the perspective of persons with disabilities, the second and third types of prevention are not terribly controversial, although there are some disability groups who might object to some forms of prenatal medical intervention. For example, some deaf families who do not regard deafness as a negative characteristic might reject prenatal cochlear implants, were such interventions available. For many persons with disabilities, though, the most disturbing type of prevention is the first: abortion. There are two reasons relating to this.

The first reason coincides with the general public controversy over abortion. People with disabilities take positions on both sides of this issue, for reasons that apply to the general populace as well as for those that are specific to persons with disabilities. On the one side, some persons with disabilities are anti-abortion for primarily disability-based reasons, including the very personal point that they might never have been born had their parents had access to prenatal screening and a legal abortion. Anecdotal accounts from adults with disabilities who were told as much by their parents validate those fears.

On the other side of the issue, many in the disability rights movement hold a strong belief in individual autonomy and support the concept of a woman's right to control her own body. Among other reasons, some disabled women and men are in favor of legal abortions because women with particular types of disabilities and medical conditions may be more likely to require late abortions of wanted pregnancies because of medical risks associated with those disabilities (Fine & Asch, 1988).

A unique disability perspective exists on both sides of the broader social debate that is largely unappreciated by the general public and by the media. It is frustrating and difficult for persons with disabilities to understand why their varied points of view on this issue are so often ignored, discounted, or simply unreported, especially when part of the debate focuses on the quality of their own lives (Morris, 1992; Saxton, 1984a, 1984b).

The other reason often cited for the widespread use of prenatal testing is due to a clash in values or beliefs about the value of life with a disability. Many in the disability rights movement and the disabled community hold a different view than does the majority of society on the effects of disability on individuals and families. The prevalent belief in many cultures is that the existence of a disability is overall a negative trait (Degener, 1990). One doesn't need to look very far to find negative images of disability in both fiction and nonfiction. Horror movies are chock-full of crazed killers who have one form of disability or another. Even fairy tales and classics read by children contain disabled villains such as Captain Hook or pathetic, helpless figures such as the little girl who can't walk until Heidi befriends her.

Generally, of course, the prevailing attitude doesn't hold that disabled people themselves are bad but that the experience of the disability contributes to a lower quality of life for the individual. This often results in a widespread assumption that if a person with a disability is experiencing difficulties, those difficulties must surely be caused by the disability and not by other factors. It also results in the disability becoming elevated to that person's predominant characteristic, as opposed to one feature out of many that define a personality.

However, people with disabilities are finding that, with advances in the availability of assistive technology, accessible environments, and appropriate social services, those widespread negative assumptions do not necessarily hold true. For many persons with a variety of disabilities, their own experiences in terms of quality of life are positive. Persons with very significant disabilities now attend regular schools, attend colleges and universities where they receive advanced degrees, find challenging jobs, get married, and live fairly normal lives.

The emerging disability rights movement is built upon the shared belief that many of the problems experienced by persons with disabilities are caused not by the disability but by the barriers that exist in society, whether they are architectural, technological, legal, or attitudinal. This is easier to see in retrospect. For example, a person who uses a wheelchair is not "confined" to the wheelchair in an accessible environment. The wheelchair is a tool, much like a pair of eyeglasses, that enables people with mobility limitations to move about wherever they please. However, until wheelchair users had the opportunity to go places freely and without assistance, a wheelchair did feel like a confining piece of equipment.

The advances in the legal rights of persons with disabilities that have taken place during the past two decades have permitted persons with disabilities to gain this new perspective about their lives. Until children with disabilities could go to their local schools and obtain the services needed to fully benefit from an education, it was easier to assume that the disabilities were the cause of the educational inequality experienced in those children's lives. Now, with a federal law mandating equality in access to education, it no longer makes sense to perceive the disability as the problem.

Why Do We Want to Prevent the Birth of Fetuses with Disabilities?

The most frequently given reasons for wanting to prevent the birth of fetuses with disabilities are to avoid negative consequences in the following areas:

economic impact on families

economic impact on society

disruption of families

quality of life of person with a disability

notions of "perfection"

It is possible to identify areas that are ripe for further inquiry by conducting an analysis of each reason. More information is needed to determine whether the assumptions behind the reasons are actually valid.

Economic Impact on Families

It is widely believed that there are disability-related costs that must be assumed by families with disabled children. While plenty of anecdotal evidence exists to support this notion, it is unclear exactly what those costs are and how predictable they are.

Some research has been conducted on the costs of raising a child with a disability. This work needs to be collected and examined to determine what the costs are associated specifically with raising a child with a disability that are not associated with raising nondisabled children. Similarly, what costs are higher for a child with a disability needs to be determined. For those special costs, what sources of support are currently available for families? Which costs must currently be borne by the families?

Economic Impact on Society

Some have pointed with alarm to the large amounts of money allocated by the government for social programs catering to persons with disabilities. The inference commonly drawn is that "prevention" through abortion will decrease those expenditures and therefore reduce public expenditures associated with disability.

The nature of public expenditures for disability needs is changing, however. In large part due to the advocacy of persons with disabilities, the purposes of many public programs are under examination. Persons with disabilities are challenging the custodial nature of many public programs and have advocated for program redesign, with the goal of providing incentives and support for employment and self-sufficiency as much as possible. Thus, new program priorities could be viewed as creating a social investment, which is paid back by the person with a disability later in life through income taxes and other types of contributions to society, both financial and other.

In addition, legislation like the Americans with Disabilities Act will have a significant impact on the American landscape, resulting in an environment with permanent fixtures that enable persons with disabilities to function like other people. It is unclear to what extent those changes will reduce the need for public expenditures that had previously served to compensate for social and architectural barriers reducing the functioning abilities of persons with disabilities.

Given the caveats above, little evidence exists to validate the assumption that abortion-based prevention will significantly reduce disability-related social costs. Research needs to be conducted to examine the following questions: To what extent are social program resources used by persons with genetic conditions? Of that group, what percentage has been reduced in recent years through genetic testing? To what extent are savings offset by public expenditures related to prenatal screening? How much money has truly been saved?

Disruption of Families

While the assumption prevails that the addition of a child with a disability to a family will be disruptive, there are anecdotal accounts supporting both sides of this question. There are accounts of families who say they have been weakened by the presence of a disabled child, as well as of those who report to have been strengthened or enriched. Presumably, there are also families who report little or no significant impact. Beyond anecdotal information, however, little solid evidence can be found either to support or refute the common view.

Without solid research into this issue, we cannot determine the impact across the many different types of families in our society. What demographic factors account for any differences in familial experiences? What other factors exist? For example, of particular importance to women is information about the extent to which mothers of disabled children are expected to disrupt their own lives in order to meet the needs of their children. Anecdotal accounts suggest that mothers assume this role far more often than do fathers.

Quality of Life

There are several possible sources of information about a person with a disability's quality of life: health and helping professionals, parents and other family members, and persons with disabilities themselves. Since quality of life is such a subjective concept, it makes sense to get information from primary sources as much as possible. This means that research into this issue should use subjects who are themselves disabled.

There is a distinction that needs to be drawn between the quality of life of the person with a disability and that of others such as family members. Many of the concerns voiced about the quality of life of family members are reflected above, and possible areas of research have been suggested. However, it is important to recognize that the experience of the person with a disability may be different than that of the other family members.

Allowing family members to report on the quality of life of the person with a disability may be misleading, because their perceptions may, at worst, be wrong or, at best, be biased by their own experiences. Thus, it is surprising and alarming that the impressions of professionals and family members have been given great credence in this regard, without any acknowledgment of their distance from the subject matter.

Little existing research refers to this subject. Further research needs to examine the subjective feelings of persons with genetically based disabilities. Subjects should be questioned about major facets of their lives (such as social life, employment, family relationships, and recreation), while persons with no disabilities should serve as a control group, responding to the same set of questions. The results of such a survey would give us much-needed information about how persons with disabilities regard their own lives.

Notions of "Perfection"

It is difficult to know whether to consider this notion seriously. However, although the goal of guaranteeing "perfection" in an offspring is not usually the stated reason for obtaining prenatal testing, it cannot be ignored. To a certain extent, this concept of perfection is tied to our notion of normalcy.

Potential research questions include: To what degree does a desire for a "normal" child factor into the decision to seek prenatal screening? What are the ethical implications of those goals? What do we mean by "perfect" or "normal"? What cultural factors contribute to different perceptions about normalcy? Are some disabilities acceptable to some groups and not to others?

The Quality of Life Dilemma

The most appealing and satisfying reason for permitting abortions based on genetic characteristics is a kind of altruism: we believe we are saving potential children from pain and harm. Other justifications, based on the economic or social interests of the family, or general societal norms, may also be present, but they do not sound as benevolent. Perhaps it is this justification that is most troublesome to disability rights activists.

What would happen to the level of social acceptance for this technology if quality of life research revealed that persons with disabilities don't share the view that the quality of their lives is significantly reduced because of their disabilities? Are the economic or social interests of others sufficient to sustain support for the technology? What would be the policy result if it were found that persons with disabilities do not report a negative subjective experience of their lives?

It is noteworthy that some of the most insistent voices questioning the rationale for prenatal screening are persons with disabilities—those whose voices most certainly deserve our attention. Persons with disabilities and their leaders are, more and more, questioning the use of prenatal screening as a response to social problems that could be resolved through other policy initiatives.

Public Perceptions of Disability

Many leaders of the disabled community (and again I emphasize persons with disabilities, as opposed to family members or professionals who often speak "for" disabled persons) have expressed concern that the widespread use of genetic testing and prenatal screening has a tendency to promote overall negative attitudes about disability. They worry that those negative attitudes result in public policies or practices that foster such problems as job discrimination, barriers to obtaining health insurance coverage, and cutbacks in public support programs (Wang, 1992).

Prenatal testing has come about during a time in which persons with disabilities and their organizations have undertaken major efforts to remove attitudinal barriers to social acceptance. They fear that the availability of prenatal testing encourages negative attitudes in several ways:

1. A general social expectation has developed that we will be able to reduce funding of programs for persons with disabilities, whether or not the actual number of persons with disabilities decreases. Prenatal screening has been promoted as beneficial because it will lead to

a reduction in the number of persons with disabilities
in society. To what extent have public policy makers,
under increasing pressure to make budget cuts, seized
upon this idea to rationalize their actions?

2. A subtle shift in perception about the causes of disability, at least in the case of genetic disabilities, results in
   the blaming of parents who "caused" a disability either by not having been screened or by having chosen
   to carry a pregnancy to term after screening revealed
   the existence of a targeted genetic trait. To what extent
   has this led to family difficulties or breakups, social
   ostracism, or other negative results?

3. There may be an increase of negative attitudes in general. In part this fear comes from language or terminology frequently used in the medical field: "bad"
   genes, "bad" babies, "defective" genes, "defective"
   babies. Do these terms extend to describe or define
   persons with disabilities? Are they "bad" people? "defective" people? They are not terms, certainly, that
   disabled people use to describe themselves. To what
   extent are negative images of disability related to those
   expressions?

4. The ability to predict the existence of a genetic condition before birth could cause increased difficulties in
   obtaining adequate medical insurance coverage for persons with disabilities. Do prenatally diagnosed conditions become "preexisting conditions"? Under current
   economic conditions, insurance companies are using a
   wide range of tactics to deny coverage to individuals
   who previously had no trouble in obtaining health insurance. To what extent has the availability of prenatal
   screening resulted in more exclusive medical insurance
   practices?

Underlying these concerns is a message that many disabled
leaders believe is implicit in the practice of abortion based on
genetic characteristics: It is better not to exist than to have a
disability. This concept is soundly rejected by the disability

rights movement, which is promoting a very different message: Most of the problems experienced by persons with disabilities are the result of intolerance, poorly conceived social programs, and environmental or communication barriers that can be removed by changes in social policy (Deegan & Brooks, 1985). These are two profoundly different perspectives on disability.

It should be pointed out that prenatal testing will never have a very significant impact on the number of persons with disabilities in the United States. It is estimated that in this country there are more than 42 million persons with a variety of disabilities—most are caused by trauma and age; relatively few are genetic in nature. Any public expectation that prenatal testing will lead to a meaningful reduction in the rates of disability in our society is quite misplaced.

Another factor that complicates the discussion is the fact that "disability" is a relative concept, as is "genetic condition." All human beings have genetic characteristics that differentiate them from other people. As our base of genetic information increases, are we at risk of creating new genetic conditions with new social stigma attached to them? Are we contracting (as opposed to expanding) the category of normal?

Where is the line drawn between a genetic characteristic and a genetic condition? At what point does a mere characteristic become an imposing condition? In a preliterate society, learning disabilities probably had much less impact on the ability of the individual to function or succeed. In a physical environment that is fully wheelchair-accessible, with low-cost and lightweight sports wheelchairs commonly available, we might not be so prone to describe wheelchair riders as "wheelchair bound" or "confined to a wheelchair." Prenatal screening cannot predict the severity of most genetic conditions, or society's perceptions of the severity, which adds further complication.

It is important to weigh these potential negative results of the availability of prenatal screening against known benefits. Thus, the benefits from prenatal screening can be more clearly defined and measured. It is also important to evaluate whether the means that are currently used to promote prenatal screening such as public service announcements, brochures, and the training of medical personnel tend to promote unacceptably negative

messages about disability. If that is the case, alternative means
or messages should be explored (Wang, 1992).

The varying perceptions of disability may partially explain
the different points of view that abound regarding the validity
of prenatal screening as a tool of public policy. If persons with
disabilities are perceived as individuals who encounter insur-
mountable difficulties in life and who place a burden on society,
prenatal screening may be regarded as a logical response. If, on
the other hand, persons with disabilities are regarded as a definable social group who have faced great oppression and stigmatization, then prenatal screening may be regarded as yet another
form of social abuse.

Conclusion

In order to evaluate the effectiveness of prenatal screening, we
must first be clear about what goals we are trying to achieve. If
we are using prenatal screening in order to attempt to protect
future human beings from experiencing a terrible quality of life,
we must be sure that there is a valid relationship between predictable genetic conditions and a negative life experience.

If we are using prenatal screening in order to attempt to resolve economic or social disadvantages that are associated with
genetic disabilities, we should first explore whether this goal
can be achieved through alternative methods and examine those
alternatives. The disability rights movement certainly agrees
that there are economic and social disadvantages associated with
disability. However, the fact that so many persons with disabilities are engaging in ordinary lives with satisfying jobs,
happy family situations, and involvement in a variety of community roles suggests that those disadvantages can be elimi-
nated without eliminating persons with disabilities.

Disability leaders have attempted to eradicate these problems
through advocacy for civil rights protections, legislation to
eradicate barriers found in the environment, programs to promote and make available adaptive technology, and more effective social support programs. Prenatal screening as a widespread social practice appears to be at odds with some of the

disability rights movement's goals, and many prominent disability leaders question its value and ethical basis (Finger, 1984).

At a minimum, prenatal testing strikes some as a technology that is proceeding without a firm basis in social policy. There are many questions about how we should proceed in an era in which proliferating information about human genetics makes matters more and more complex. We surely need to include the perspectives of the disabled community more fully in our research and exploration of policy options. The disability community is willing to join in the dialogue.

BIBLIOGRAPHY

DEEGAN, M. J., & Brooks, N. A. (1985). *Women and disability: The double handicap.* New Brunswick, NJ: Transaction.

DEGENER, T. (1990). Female self-determination between feminist claims and 'voluntary' eugenics, between 'rights' and ethics. *Issues in Reproductive and Genetic Engineering, 3*(2), 87–99.

FINE, M., & Asch, A. (Eds.). (1988). *Women with disabilities: Essays in psychology, culture and politics.* Philadelphia: Temple University Press.

FINGER, A. (1984). Claiming all of our bodies: Reproductive rights and disabilities. In R. Arditti, R. Duelli-Klein, & S. Minden (Eds.), *Test-tube women: What future for motherhood?* Boston: Routledge/Kegan.

MORRIS, J. (1992). Tyrannies of perfection. *New Internationalist, 233,* 16.

SAXTON, M. (1984a). Born and unborn: Implications of the reproductive technologies for people with disabilities. In R. Arditti, R. Duelli-Klein, & S. Minden (Eds.), *Test-tube women: What future for motherhood?* Boston: Routledge/Kegan.

SAXTON, M. (1984b). The implications of 'choice' for people with disabilities. *Women Wise, The N.H. Feminist Health Center Quarterly,* Winter.

WANG, C. (1992). Culture, meaning and disability: Injury prevention campaigns and the production of stigma. *Social Science Medicine, 35*(9), 1093–1102.

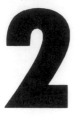

Philosophical, Ethical, and Legal Perspectives

The first three chapters in this part set forth the philosophical foundations and complex ethical questions raised by reproductive genetic testing. Mary Mahowald examines the concept of gender justice and relates this to different versions of feminism and a care-based ethic. She presents alternative theoretical approaches not only to the use of gender-neutral language but to the entire range of issues in reproductive genetic testing considered in this book. Is it possible to neutralize gender issues when dealing with reproduction, since women, out of necessity (at least in part due to biology) will be more involved in the benefits and the burdens associated with reproductive genetic testing? Mahowald proposes a strategy for promoting the goal of gender justice in this area.

Ruth Faden examines whether and to what extent women are morally obliged to seek reproductive genetic testing. Should prospective mothers (and fathers) seek or accept testing? Should prospective mothers seek or accept therapeutic interventions based on the results of testing? What in the absence of therapy should prospective mothers do when a fetus is identified as having "a problem"? She concludes that, with rare exceptions, there is no requirement in mothering (or parenting) to seek or accept testing if the only actions facilitated by such testing are abortion, selective conception, or remaining childless. Patricia King's commentary suggests that such questions remain difficult to resolve because there is a lack of adequate theoretical basis for understanding the structure and functioning of the family, especially the parent–child relationship. She concludes that a revised framework for understanding this relationship is needed to acknowledge the diversity of women and their families so that ethical decisions are made in context, rather than in abstraction.

The next two chapters bridge the gap between ethics and legal issues. Alta Charo and Karen Rothenberg raise the legal implications of creating the standard of the "good mother" in the context of reproductive genetic testing. They pose the question that even if there is support for moral accountability, is it ever appropriate to hold a woman legally accountable for her reproductive genetic testing decisions? They argue that legal accountability adds little to the already significant emotional and financial forces constraining reproductive choices. They further reject the notion that there are objective legal standards to measure those lives worth living and those not. An analysis of the political, legal, and ethical underpinnings of individual rights and community interests leads to the conclusion that justifications to manipulate women's reproductive decisions are fatally flawed.

Following this analysis, Ellen Wright Clayton describes the present state of the law on the provision of genetic services, access to abortion services, wrongful birth and wrongful life actions, and the governmental response to reproductive genetic testing. While some social forces have increased access to testing, others have attempted to limit testing by failing to provide funds, by forbidding lawsuits, and by limiting access to abortion. What are the underlying forces that are resulting in conflicting public policy and law and how can these differences be resolved? In the light of these legal ambiguities and inconsistencies, Clayton encourages a more coherent approach to respond to such issues in the future.

4 Reproductive Genetics and Gender Justice

MARY B. MAHOWALD

In recent years, the use of gender-neutral terminology has become commonplace. At times the practice is awkward, as when a writer or speaker avoids generic terms that are also used exclusively for males. "Human" or "person" then replaces "man," and "he or she" is often used instead of merely "he." Despite the awkwardness, this practice may have the positive effect of reminding readers or listeners of a topic's applicability to women as well as to men, or vice versa. Ethical support for the practice stems from the view that men and women should be given equal attention to ensure that sexism does not surface or prevail. Sexism is definable as unjust or unequal treatment of the members of one sex in comparison with the other.[1] Like racism and classism, it is generally considered a moral wrong.

The position supported here is that the tendency to consider certain issues in a gender-neutral manner is misguided and unlikely to achieve its presumed end of gender justice. I argue that consideration of gender differences, as well as of the differences among individuals, is crucial to that goal and consistent with an ethic of care as well as of justice. While I focus on reproductive genetics to illustrate various points, my position is applicable to other issues as well. Poverty, aging, and violence, for example, all involve a gender-specific component in their impact on people's lives.

To develop my argument I examine the concept of gender justice and relate this to different versions of feminism and a care-based ethic. I thus present alternative theoretical approaches not only to the use of gender-neutral language but to the entire range of issues in reproductive genetic testing considered in this book. My goal is to prod the reader to come to his or her own conclusions about the meaning and desirability of gender justice and its applicability to issues of reproductive genetics. I also propose a modest strategy for promoting the goal of gender justice. Preliminarily, I offer examples of ways in which current discussions illustrate the misguided tendency to use gender-neutral language.

Gender-Neutral Language in Reproductive Genetics

Reproductive endocrinologists write about infertile *couples* even when it is clear that one partner is infertile and the other is not.[2] Infertility, it is claimed, is a problem of couples rather than of individuals because both male and female partners are essential contributors to the reproductive process. Similarly, prenatal testing is generally offered to couples rather than individuals despite the fact that the main modalities of testing are performed on the female partner (Bonnicksen, 1992, p. S5; Lippman, 1991, pp. 38–39). Pregnancy terminations and fetal therapies in response to prenatal diagnoses are also discussed in the context of couples, although neither procedure requires participation or risk by the male partner (Elias & Annas, 1987, pp. 121–142).

Oftentimes parental rights and responsibilities are considered generically—as if mothers and fathers are equally involved in childbearing and childrearing (Blustein, 1979, pp. 115–119). Gamete donors are also assumed equal despite the fact that the risk and discomfort of ova donation is not present in sperm donation (Jones, 1992, pp. 753–754). It has even been suggested that the rights of sperm donors are, or should be, equal to those of women who not only provide ova but undergo artificial insemination, gestation, and childbirth.[3]

Gender differences among researchers in genetics[4] and clinical geneticists[5] (Pencarinha, Bell, Edwards, & Best, 1992) are rarely if ever noted despite the gender imbalance that is evident between those in the more powerful, prestigious, and highly paid positions, and those at the lower end of the spectrum. The writings of Dorothy Wertz and John Fletcher, along with Nancy Zare and her colleagues, are welcome exceptions to this trend (Wertz & Fletcher, 1989, 1992; Zare, Sorenson, & Heeren, 1984). Gender differences are also rarely noted among those who have primary care responsibility for those affected by genetic conditions. By far, the majority of these are women whose primary care of children, the ill, and the elderly has led to the phenomenon that Diana Pearce characterizes as "the feminization of poverty" (1978, p. 28).

Most if not all of the preceding examples suggest the possibility of injustice toward women. It is women whose bodies undergo discomfort and risk in the course of prenatal testing, and women whose physical and emotional energies are more likely to be consumed by the exigencies of care for those who are genetically disabled. With regard to gender differences involving genetic conditions, however, the opposite point may be made. X-linked diseases, for instance, mainly affect men; women have the preempting advantage of a second X chromosome. It is women, nonetheless, who as carriers of X-linked diseases bear the onus of having "given" their affected sons the disease. In addition, some genetic conditions (for example, cystic fibrosis, Down syndrome) generally cause infertility in affected men but not in affected women. Although men never face health risks due to pregnancy, pregnancy presents a particular health threat to women affected by certain genetic diseases (for example, cystic fibrosis and sickle-cell anemia) (Lemke, 1992, pp. 213–214; Koshy & Burd, 1991, pp. 587–590).

All of these empirical differences between women and men involving reproductive genetics are ethically problematic, and largely so because justice or equality is often construed as an ethical demand to treat all individuals in the same way. Clearly, it is not possible to treat women and men in the same way with regard to reproduction. One cannot, for example, retrieve ova from women as easily as sperm are retrieved from men. One cannot perform abortions or fetal therapies on men. So if there is such a thing as gender justice in reproductive genetics, it must mean something different than treating men and women in the same way.

Gender Justice and Different Versions of Feminism

Gender and sex are commonly distinguished on the grounds of the difference between socialization and biology, or nurture and nature. Sex is biologically determined, and gender, although usually based on sex assignment, is established through socialization (Jaggar, 1983, p. 112).[6] Sex generally refers to physical characteristics, whether genetic, anatomic, or functional; gender refers to behavior. The differences between males and females and between men and women, which are key to understanding sex and gender, are commonly seen in terms of privation or negation. For example, the female *lacks* testes and penis; the male is *unable* to bear or nurse a child. To be male, then, is not to be female, and to be a woman is not to be a man.

Furthermore, differences are commonly construed as connoting inequality.[7] This construct is valid when its reference point is the same for the differences being compared, so that one difference represents more or less of the other—for example, when one person's income or education is compared with another's income or education. The construct is invalid when the reference point is not the same because there is then no common basis for comparison—for example, when one person's maleness is compared with another person's femaleness. Differences do not imply inequality if they represent incomparable factors, that is, factors that have no common reference point.

Gender injustice, sexism, or sex inequality does not necessarily occur when men or women are regarded or treated differently but when they are regarded or treated in a manner by which the essential differences of one sex are interpreted as implying their inferiority to the other, and they are treated accordingly.[8] The reference point to which women are typically compared is men, rather than the common humanness in which men and women participate equally. In *The Second Sex* Simone de Beauvoir describes this phenomenon as one in which "man defines woman not in herself but as relative to him," that is, as "the Other" who is "the incidental, the inessential as opposed to the essential" (1971, p. xvi). In contrast, gender justice occurs when men and women alike are judged according to the standard of their common humanness, respecting the differences that they embody as gendered individuals without imputing inferiority to one or the other on that basis.

Inequality, even when validly established, is not necessarily unjust. It is not unjust, for example, that older people typically have a wider range of experiences and a more extended life span than younger people. Nor is it unjust that some people are more talented, more intelligent, more attractive, or more athletically gifted than others. In comparing unequal distributions of such factors among individuals, H. Tristram Engelhardt suggests that such differences are due to failures of fortune rather than fairness (1986, p. 342). It is unfortunate, then, that some people are disabled while others are fully abled, but it is not unfair that this is so. Engelhardt would probably not claim that it is unfortunate for women that they are not born male; yet such a statement would be empirically supportable on grounds that women are more likely than men to be poor and dependent on the health care system for themselves and others, and less likely than men to be well-educated or to find positions of power and prestige (Mahowald, 1993, pp. 39n. 1, 219–220).

Engelhardt's distinction between what is unfortunate and what is unfair is based on the fact that no one is responsible for the differences that create inequality. But this alone fails to address what is done or not done about the differences by those who, arguably at least, have responsibility subsequent to that creation. Different concepts of justice may be introduced to validate alternative means of responding to differences. The alternatives range from procedure-based libertarian theories such as Robert Nozick's, through theories that attempt to combine elements of both libertarian and egalitarian reasoning such as John Rawls's, to idealistically egalitarian theories such as Karl Marx's. Each of those involves a different view of gender justice and is thus relatable to different versions of feminism.

A libertarian theory of justice gives priority to the liberty of individuals in choosing procedural mechanisms for the distribution of goods. The economic system thus supported is capitalistic, individualistic, and rights-centered. Self-interest is the force that motivates individuals to freely enter, continue, and withdraw from socioeconomic arrangements, whose rules they are bound—by virtue of their agreement—to observe. As Nozick paraphrases Marx, the libertarian criterion for decisions regarding distribution is: "From each as they choose, to each as they are chosen" (1974, p. 160).[9] This concept of justice is essentially procedural rather than substantive. Depending on differences in the individuals whose liberty is equally respected under the aegis of the theory, the material gaps between them are inevitably widened through maximization of individual liberty in a laissez-faire environment. Nozick's dictum involves no restriction of the content of one's choices; it therefore permits racist, sexist, and classist choices as well as choices that are morally praiseworthy—so long as such choices are consistent with procedural fairness.

In reproductive genetics, both libertarian and liberal feminist arguments have been applied to specific issues. From a libertarian perspective such as Engelhardt's, for example, as long as a woman can pay for prenatal diagnosis and treatment, and is fully informed about the risks she freely undertakes, reproductive genetic testing is ethically justified. Since the emphasis is on *individual* liberty, however, the tendency to treat those issues in the context of couples rather than individuals is inappropriate. Lori Andrews recognizes the inappropriateness when she argues that a feminist position on a woman's right to control the disposition of her own body is contradicted by feminists who oppose the rights of individual women to provide ova or gestation in exchange for money (1988, p. 82).

Liberalism and liberal feminism are also associated with an emphasis on individual liberty. However, liberal feminism defends an equality of opportunity that reduces the inequality that is theoretically justifiable in a libertarian system. Some of the implications of the liberal feminist position are clear, but some are not. It seems clear, for example, that women as well as men have a right to basic health care and to an environment that is free of contaminants that might damage their own and their offspring's health. It is not clear whether equality of opportunity requires the availability of prenatal counseling and intervention for all women. The extent to which government is obliged to pay for the reproductive health care of those who cannot pay for it themselves is a matter on which liberal feminists are likely to disagree. Some would support a minimal level of government subsidies, leaning closer to a libertarian approach; others would support a maximal level, with more egalitarian implications.

Rawls's theory of justice is an effort to combine liberal and egalitarian considerations. His first principle of justice incorporates the liberal's emphasis: Individual liberty should be limited only to the extent that it is necessary to ensure the same liberty for others. Rawls's second principle of justice expresses the egalitarian component of his theory: Social and economic inequalities should be arranged so that they benefit the least advantaged in a situation of equality of opportunity for all (1971, p. 302). In *Justice, Gender, and the Family*, Susan Moller Okin endorses those principles of justice, but criticizes Rawls for assuming that family constructs are just (1989, p. 97). She develops a contrasting liberal feminist account using data illustrating that the inherently patriarchal structure of the family is unjust, and that injustice toward women is often triggered by family-related practices and attitudes.

Okin's theoretical critique extends to "false gender neutrality" in language as well as in action. She insists on paying attention to gender differences that might provoke injustice, even while arguing for an ideal of a "genderless family." Unlike most philosophers, she offers specific recommendations: "Because children are borne by women but can (and, I contend, should) be raised by both parents equally, policies relating to pregnancy and birth should be quite distinct from those relating to parenting. Pregnancy and childbirth, to whatever varying extent they require leave from work, should be regarded as temporarily disabling conditions like any others, and employers should be mandated to provide leave for all such conditions" (1989, p. 176). The same recommendations are applicable to issues that arise in reproductive genetic testing. For example, because men do not undergo the risk and discomfort of prenatal diagnosis, the time and cost of the procedures should not be borne by women alone but should be shared with men either directly (as couples paying for services) or indirectly (through employer or government coverage).

Critics of liberal feminism may focus either on its liberal component or its feminist component. The liberal component has been critiqued for its tendency to treat individuals atomistically, emphasizing rights rather than relationships and responsibilities.[10] The feminist component has been critiqued by feminists themselves for subscribing to an essentially male model of rationality and autonomy. One of the results of this subscription, according to Alison Jaggar, is a "normative dualism" with regard to our evaluation of the relationship between mind and body (1983, p. 40). In a society that generally views activities of the mind as superior to those of the body, women are likely to be less esteemed because gestation, birth, and early nurturance of children tie them more to physical than to mental activities. Jaggar also maintains that a liberal feminist emphasis on individual autonomy provides an inadequate account of moral goodness. Beyond respect for others' choices, the ends we pursue as individuals and as a society ought to promote the survival of humans and their thriving (Tong, 1989, p. 37).

The normative dualism that Jaggar criticizes is apparent in attitudes and practices with regard to genetic diseases that are mainly associated with mental retardation. For example, the desire to avoid the birth of a child with Down syndrome is the most common reason for women to undergo prenatal testing (Elias & Annas, 1987, p. 84). Although specific physical findings and other medical problems are often associated with Down syndrome, the principal problem the condition presents is mental retardation. Jaggar's insistence that other values besides respect for autonomy should be considered in our moral judgments is also applicable to reproductive genetics. The justification for nondirective counseling, for example, is primarily based on respect for the client's autonomy. Jaggar and other socialist feminists would argue that considerations of beneficence and social justice are relevant to the counseling situation as well.

Like Angus Clarke, who describes nondirective counseling as "the Holy Grail," socialist feminists are concerned not only about women's right to abortion but also about "the social pressures that may be exerted on couples, and especially on women, to terminate a pregnancy thought to be affected by a genetic disorder" (Clarke, 1991, p. 1000). They would further agree with Clarke's concerns about the implications of prenatal diagnosis for "society as a whole, with long-term repercussions for the status of, and provision for, the mentally and physically handicapped" (p. 998). Consideration of these repercussions through attention to differences between individuals as well as groups is crucial to the goal of social equality.

Communitarian or socialist thinkers are the principal critics of liberal feminism (Tong, 1989, pp. 32–37). Communitarians tend to emphasize familial or affective relationships, while socialists emphasize political relationships and the importance of equality as a social goal. A communitarian ideology may be reinforced by the care models of moral reasoning that Carol Gilligan (1982) and Nel Noddings (1984) have developed. Gilligan's studies indicate that women are more likely than men to base their ethical decisions on considerations of care rather than justice. Noddings argues that ethical caring is based on the inclination of women to care for their offspring. Although both models are based on women's experiences, some feminists are critical of them because they may promote exploitation of women's natural propensity to care for others (Sherwin, 1992, pp. 49–57). Because women are the primary caregivers, both formally and informally, of persons affected by genetic conditions, possibilities for exploitation are evident in that context. If caring behavior were as esteemed and rewarded as behavior based on a justice model of reasoning, exploitation would probably be avoided.

Jaggar distinguishes between socialist and Marxist feminism on the grounds of the primacy given to the oppression of women (1983, p. 12). Marxist feminists, she claims, see women's oppression as an expression of the fundamental economic oppression that separates the bourgeoisie from the proletariat. As Marx put it, the degree of humaneness that is evident in the relationship between men and women is an indicator of the progress in humaneness of the entire society (Tucker, 1972, p. 69). However, the goal of correcting injustice or inequality between men and women is subordinate to the goal of overcoming economic oppression between capitalists and workers.

In contrast, socialist feminists see the oppression of women as the primordial social injustice, with other forms of oppression stemming from this. Overcoming gender inequality is thus central to the socialist feminist agenda.

Socialist feminist concerns about reproductive genetics target the problem of access to genetic services, treatment options, and information. Admittedly, it is difficult if not impossible to disentangle the influence of cultural values from the influence of socioeconomic determinants on access to prenatal counseling and interventions. Among those who undergo counseling, however, poor women and women of color are clearly underrepresented (Reynolds, Puck, & Robinson, 1974, p. 180; Nsiah-Jefferson & Hall, 1989, pp. 93–95). They are even more underrepresented, in fact comparatively absent, in the ranks of those who seek and obtain expensive reproductive technologies such as in vitro fertilization and surrogate gestation (Nsiah-Jefferson & Hall, 1989, pp. 108–111). Poor women and women of color are more likely to be numbered among those who provide genetic services through their own bodies (such as through egg "donation" and commercial surrogacy) and through their own labor (such as through employment among the less prestigious and less rewarded ranks of health care workers) (Mahowald, 1993, pp. 25, 102–104).

Even in cases where genetic information is provided, the options for poor women are limited through legislation that precludes the possibility of pregnancy termination for those unable to pay. For individuals who cannot terminate the gestation of an abnormal fetus because of the cost of the procedure, prenatal diagnosis may not be worth the risk and discomfort that it entails. For those who have no coverage through insurance or government reimbursement plans, even the advantage of ascertaining that the fetus has no genetic abnormalities may not be worth the cost of prenatal diagnosis. Whether considering the option of prenatal diagnosis or pregnancy termination, the onus of the procedure falls on women rather than men.

From a socialist feminist standpoint, society and individuals alike are morally bound to take account of this discrepancy and attempt to reduce it. Minimizing the cost and risk of the procedures and maximizing access to them would constitute such an attempt. One way of reducing the gender gap in this regard would be requiring the partners of women who undergo prenatal diagnosis and pregnancy termination to pay for the procedure. The spread of the feminization of poverty must be checked on several fronts in order to provide women with an equal balance of health prospects in comparison with men.

Socialist feminists are also concerned with the implications of genetic testing for the availability of jobs and progress in employment. The U.S. Supreme Court's decision in the *Johnson Controls* case is reassuring with regard to the legality of employment practices that restrict women's opportunities because of their reproductive capacity.[11] But that decision does not negate the tendency of employers to be influenced by such concerns and act in ways that are discriminatory towards women. Insurance practices are another area in which gender discrimination relevant to reproductive genetics is sometimes practiced (Natowicz, Alper, & Alper, 1992, p. 467).

As more and more genetic information is obtained through the success of the Human Genome Project, the possibilities for discrimination increase. Socialist feminism rejects such practices through its critique of the capitalistic ideology that supports them. Without subscribing to a totalitarian system, social feminism supports limitation of individual freedom to promote social equality. Lest this be construed as a radical proposal, it should be recognized that American society already endorses anticapitalistic or socialistic measures such as a graduated income tax, government subsidies to farmers, and welfare payments for the poor. Government regulation intended to avoid genetic discrimination based on gender would also involve curtailment of liberty for the sake of equality. To be effective, however, such regulation needs to take explicit account of the gender-based differences that lead to discrimination. To the extent that regulations limit liberty to promote equality, they are socialist in their orientation.

Admittedly, the term socialist has been in disrepute since the demise of the Soviet Union and other officially socialist or Marxist states. However, the term itself is not a crucial label for the critique of individualism and liberalism that many feminists support. What is essential to the critique is that it starts

with a concept of human beings not as isolated individuals but
as individuals whose meaning and reality are definable and sus-
tainable only in the context of their relationships to others.
This emphasis on relationships is common to socialist feminism, communitarian versions of feminism, and to the ethics of
care or caring that Gilligan and Noddings have developed.
Noddings claims the relationship between mother and child as
ethically paradigmatic, and argues for a broader application of
the care embodied in that relationship (1984, pp. 43, 79–81). Gilligan bases her model of moral reasoning on studies of girls
and women confronting ethical dilemmas in their own lives
(1982, p. 3). Women, she found, typically reached their decisions through consideration of responsibilities derived from relationships to others rather than consideration of their own or
others' rights as individuals. They were more likely than men
to be influenced by concerns of caring toward those with whom
they had established ties than by concerns of justice toward
those they did not know.

Wertz has examined whether Gilligan's distinction between
justice and care models of reasoning is supported by studies
of providers of genetic counseling (1993, p. 85). The justice
model encapsulates the traditional approaches to ethics that (for
the most part male) philosophers have pursued for centuries.
Whether those approaches appeal to consequences through utilitarianism or to a priori rules developed through deontological
theories, they maintain that moral decisions must be based on
abstract, impartial, and universalizable principles. In contrast,
the care-based reasoning that women tend to practice involves
concreteness, partiality, and particularity. Wertz's work, along
with a recent study by Pencarinha (1992), suggests that women
who work as genetic counselors do not fit neatly into either of
Gilligan's models of moral reasoning.

Nonetheless, Wertz maintains that gender is "the single most
important determinant of ethical decision-making" among doctoral level medical geneticists around the world (1993, p. 81).
Although the majority of those surveyed were committed to
nondirective counseling, men were 2 to 13 times (depending
on the country) more likely to be directive. The women (35%
of the respondents) in Wertz and Fletcher's study were also

more likely than the men to emphasize client autonomy and to express concern about the families of their clients (Wertz & Fletcher, 1992, p. 236). Their emphasis on the client's autonomy, often expressed in phrases like "the right to know" and "the right to decide," reflects the philosophical tradition of ethics that care-based thinkers generally reject. The concern about families, however, reflects the critique of individualism with which care-based thinkers agree. This critique is the point at which a care ethic and communitarian or socialist versions of feminism converge through their emphasis on relationships.

Pencarinha and her colleagues compared the ethical decision-making of masters level genetic counselors and doctoral level (M.D. or Ph.D.) medical geneticists in the United States. In contrast to the medical geneticists, the majority of whom are men, 94% of genetic counselors are women. The genetic counselors in Pencarinha's study primarily stressed the autonomy of their individual clients as their guiding ethical norm. They were even more likely than medical geneticists to be nondirective, to respect client confidentiality even in cases where nondisclosure might threaten others' welfare, and to refer clients to another center for sex selection (1992, pp. 23–28). To the extent that their respect for the autonomy of individual clients overrode concerns for other family members, genetic counselors in Pencarinha's study departed from a care-based model of moral reasoning and illustrated traditional ethical (Kantian) reasoning even more than did the women in Wertz and Fletcher's study. Attributing this priority to autonomy is consistent with liberal and libertarian versions of feminism.

Toward a Feminist Care-Based Ethic

Just as men and women are not necessarily incompatible or unequal because they are different, a care-based ethic and a justice ethic are not necessarily incompatible or unequally valid because they are different. Gilligan suggests that there are liabilities to either approach. The potential error of a justice focus, she says, is "its latent egocentrism, the tendency to confuse one's perspective with an objective standpoint or truth, the temptation to define others in one's own terms by putting oneself in their place." The liability of a focus on care is that it tends "to forget that one has terms, creating a tendency to enter into another's perspective and to see oneself as 'selfless' by defining oneself in others' terms" (1987, p. 31). Historically, those liabilities have given rise to two common distortions of justice and care. In an ethic of justice the distortion is that human is equated with male; in an ethic of care the distortion is the equation of care with self-sacrifice. The liabilities are avoided and the distortions are corrected in an ethic that incorporates both justice and care. According to Pencarinha's study, women who work as genetic counselors illustrate elements of both justice and care.

Genetic counselors may be particularly inclined to emphasize client autonomy because they recognize that the lives of their clients, most of whom are women, are affected more than are their male partners' by decisions involving reproductive genetics. They may be more inclined to recognize this gender difference because most of them are women. This practice is feminist to the extent that it promotes or is intended to promote gender justice.

To the extent that genetic counselors honor women's autonomy, they also support the reasons for which individual women make their reproductive decisions. If Gilligan is right, these reasons tend to be based on the complex set of caring relationships that each woman bears to others. Maximizing women's autonomy in decisions about reproductive genetics is thus a way of maximizing caring. Because women in our society are in several ways less powerful than men (for example, economically), maximizing their autonomy is also a way of promoting equality or reducing inequality between them and men. Gender justice, implemented through support for the autonomy of those most affected by reproductive decisions, is a means, perhaps even an indispensable means, through which to realize an ethic based on caring.

While questioning whether either orientation is, in and of itself, adequate from a moral point of view, Marilyn Friedman maintains that care and justice are compatible (1987, p. 105). If justice means giving people their due, it demands determination of what constitutes due care for each. The application of this concept to reproductive genetics is obvious: the practitioner must recognize and respond to different needs or interests on the part of each client. At times the needs of different clients are at odds with each other, such as when the counselor learns that the assumed father of a child is not genetically related to that child. Wertz's and Pencarinha's studies show that most genetic counselors believe that the confidentiality of the child's mother should be upheld in such situations. Depending on the risk that not knowing entails for others, however, nondisclosure may be morally unjust. A caring ethic is thus different from an ethic of health care that focuses solely on the client because it involves care for all of those affected by the carer's decisions. A *just* caring ethic requires efforts to distribute burdens and benefits in an equitable manner.

The focus on women that constitutes the subject matter of this book is a means of overcoming the mistaken tendency to treat reproductive genetics as if it were gender-neutral. This focus is appropriately represented through a predominance of women authors. Although some men grasp and communicate the significance of women's role in reproductive genetics better than do some women, women know better than men what women experience. Accordingly, feminists have argued recently for the necessity of a feminist standpoint in decisions and policies that particularly affect women. Sara Ruddick describes such a standpoint as "an engaged vision of the world opposed and superior to dominant ways of thinking" (1989, p. 129). The rationale for a feminist standpoint is both ethical and epistemological. In reproductive genetics, ethical arguments for a feminist standpoint are based on the fact that women's bodies and lives are generally more affected than men's by reproductive decisions. As abortion legislation illustrates, this gives them the more compelling right to determine the outcome in situations of conflict.

The epistemological argument for a feminist standpoint involves what Donna Haraway affirms as "the embodied nature of all vision" (1988, p. 581). Haraway regards the impartial standpoint of traditional ethics as neither feasible nor desirable. The alternative she proposes is "a doctrine of embodied objectivity," which involves "partial, locatable, critical knowledges sustaining the possibility of webs of connections called solidarity in politics and shared conversations in epistemology" (1988, p. 584). Only through such partial perspectives, she claims, can we approach objectivity.

A feminist standpoint may draw on any of the diverse versions of feminism because all of these involve a remedial emphasis on women. In fact, the enrichment of perspectives that their inclusion involves can only be maximized by including representatives of diverse feminisms. Women are also distinguishable from one another by class, race, and sexual orientation, and by size, age, politics, religion, and profession. Thus, while they belong to the nondominant group by gender, some women belong to the dominant group by race or class. Just as women have a privileged epistemological status vis-à-vis men, the same is true for women of color vis-à-vis white women, and clients or patients vis-à-vis the professionals (women or men) who treat or counsel them. Moreover, because women as individuals are not definable through any collection of categorical designations, the rationale that underlies a feminist standpoint must be extended to a recognition of each woman as a unique individual. To promote gender justice for all women, individual differences as well as gender and other group-based differences must be taken into account.

How, practically, can so many differences be fully considered in order to effect just policies and decision-making in reproductive genetics? An honest answer to this question is "They can't." This does not imply, however, that it is useless to consider the differences and to attempt to minimize the inadequacy of their consideration. Accordingly, I wish to conclude with the recommendation of a single, modest guideline that the preceding discussion suggests with regard to decisions and policies in reproductive genetics. It is simple, obvious, and demanding: Listen to women.

Aside from the fact that women may have a different moral voice than men, they have a different role, experience, and responsibility with regard to reproduction. The only way to adequately consider those differences is to learn about them from women themselves. Legislative and policy-making bodies that address issues in reproductive genetics need more, and more diverse, women in their ranks. Adequate representation of women may be an unachievable goal because women are so diverse as individuals and as participants in other groups. Nonetheless, their representation could surely be improved by specific measures intended to facilitate that. For example, if we valued the participation of poor women enough to pay them and ensure that their income would not be threatened by their participation, we might increase our socioeconomic representation. If we were willing to challenge the political pragmatism or homophobia that has triggered the exclusion of lesbians and homosexuals from participation, we might also broaden our representation. Participation of more and more diverse women, as well as participation of nondominant groups of men, is a plausible goal, although one not managed without cost and effort.

If broader representation were implemented as a means of reducing the inevitable "nearsightedness" of the dominant class or classes, the different voices of women and minorities would certainly be heard in decisions and policies made about reproductive genetics.[12] They would be heard as practitioners and clients, as policy makers, and as teachers of those who belong to the dominant class. Such representation would also mean that tokenism, such as having one woman or African American serve on a policy-making committee, is not enough, particularly when the group's decisions disproportionately affect those who are not dominant. When a single individual represents several nondominant groups, her voice and vote should count additionally for each of the groups represented.

Unfortunately, there are some situations in which too few nondominant persons are available to provide fair representation. For example, very few of those trained as genetic counselors are persons of color (Pencarinha et al., 1992, p. 21). Self-consciousness about one's inevitable nearsightedness is demanded of the dominant individuals who render the representation disproportionate. With regard to gender differences, such self-consciousness involves acknowledgment of a possible sexist bias even on the part of those who consider themselves free of such bias. As Virginia Warren observes, "Sexist ethics would never appear sexist [even to the person practicing it]. It would be clothed in a cloak of neutrality because favoring some group or position would be unthinkable" (1989, p. 74). A similar observation applies to groups distinguishable by race, class, mental or physical ability, and sexual orientation. To those who consider themselves capable of total impartiality, inclusion of others' perspectives is unnecessary.

Listening to other women is as important for women as listening to women is for men. Such listening is often demanding because it requires the listeners to refrain from exercising their own powers of speech temporarily. It also requires psychological openness to new and critical ideas, that is, a kind of intellectual humility. At times, the learning that comes from listening changes our views of ourselves as well as of others, but even as we grow through listening, so do the others. A necessary means to continuing the growth is to keep on listening.

Listening to women, and learning from and acting on what we hear from women, constitutes an indispensable means of promoting gender justice in reproductive genetics. While different versions of feminism support different degrees and concepts of social equality, they concur about the importance of listening to women's different voices.

ACKNOWLEDGMENTS

Research for this paper has been supported by grant #HG00641–01 from the National Center for Human Genome Research of the National Institutes of Health. I also wish to acknowledge helpful comments from Amy Lemke, co-investigator, and Karin Bowman, coordinator, for this grant.

NOTES

1. The *Oxford English Dictionary* (1989) defines sexism as "the assumption that one sex is superior to the other and the resultant discrimination practiced against members of the supposed inferior sex, esp. by men against women"; *Webster's New World Dictionary* (1984) defines it as "the economic exploitation and social domination of members of one sex by the other, specif. of women by men." Both definitions suggest that the inequality or injustice of sexism involves the inappropriate use of power. For a critical consideration of power and a criterion for distinguishing between its moral and immoral uses, see Mahowald, 1993, pp. 256–59.

2. Howard Jones, for example, who with Georgianna Jones developed the first successful in vitro clinic in the United States, maintains that "physicians should realize that they are treating not infertility, but a couple—two individuals— who are infertile" (Jones, 1992, p. 751).

3. *In re* Baby M 217 N.J. Super 313 (1987).
4. Women comprise approximately 21% of genetics researchers who have been awarded grants by the National Center for Human Genome Research of the National Institutes of Health (Training Grants Active on 8/1/92), National Center for Human Genome Research.
5. Of 677 doctoral level medical geneticists from 18 countries who responded to a survey by Wertz and Fletcher, 65% were men. The women in this group were more likely to have a Ph.D. and less likely to have an M.D. (Wertz & Fletcher, 1992, p. 234). Of 199 masters level genetic counselors in the United States surveyed by Pencarinha et al., only 6.5% were men (1992, p. 21).
6. As Jaggar remarks, however, if "we acknowledge human biology, including sexual biology, as created partly by society, and if we acknowledge human society as responding to human biology, we lose the clarity of the distinctions between sex and gender" (1983, p. 112).
7. A classical exemplar of this construct is Thomas Aquinas, who maintains that in the first state of nature, that is, nature as created by God, "there would have been some inequality, at least as regards sex, because generation depends upon diversity of sex" ("On the First Man," Q. 96, cited in Mahowald, 1992, p. 284).
8. This point, along with a concept of equality as a social ideal and guidelines consistent with gender justice, is developed in chapter 1 and applied to a variety of issues involving women and children in Mahowald, 1993.
9. One wonders whether Nozick's use of the gender-neutral "they," in the light of its grammatical incorrectness, is deliberate.
10. Some critics argue that the liberal's emphasis on the priority of the individual constitutes an impediment to human community. Jean Bethke Elshtain, for example, claims that "there is no way to create real communities out of an aggregate of 'freely' choosing adults" (1986, p. 442).
11. *Automobile Workers v. Johnson Controls*, 499 U.S. 187 (1991).
12. In another article I have called this concept "proportionate representation," and have applied it more generally to issues in bioethics. See my "On Treatment of Myopia: Feminist Standpoint Theory and Bioethics," in Susan Wolf, ed., *Feminism and Bioethics* (Oxford University Press, forthcoming).

BIBLIOGRAPHY

ANDREWS, L. B. (1988). Feminism revisited: Fallacies and policies in the surrogacy debate. *Logos, 9*, 81–96.

BLUSTEIN, J. (1979). Child rearing and family interests. In O. O'Neill & W. Ruddick (Eds.), *Having children: Philosophical and legal reflections on parenthood* (pp. 115–122). New York: Oxford University Press.

BONNICKSEN, A. (1992). Genetic diagnosis of human embryos. *Hastings Center Report, 22*(4), S5-S11.

CLARKE, A. (1991). Is non-directive genetic counselling possible? *Lancet,* *338,* 998-1001.

DE BEAUVOIR, S. (1971). *The second sex* (H. M. Parshley Trans. and Ed.). New York: Knopf.

ELIAS, S., & Annas, G. J. (1987). *Reproductive genetics and the law.* Chicago: Year Book Medical Publishers.

ELSHTAIN, J. B. (1986). Feminism, family, and community. *Dissent, 29,* 442–449.

ENGLEHARDT, H. T. (1986). *The foundations of bioethics.* New York: Oxford University Press.

FRIEDMAN, M. (1987). Beyond caring: The de-moralization of gender. In M. Hanen & K. Nielsen (Eds.), *Science, morality and feminist theory* (pp. 87–110). Calgary, Alberta: University of Calgary Press.

GILLIGAN, C. (1982). *In a different voice: Psychological theory and women's development.* Cambridge, MA: Harvard University Press.

GILLIGAN, C. (1987). Moral orientation and moral development. In E. F. Kittay & D. T. Meyers (Eds.), *Women and moral theory* (pp. 19–33). Totowa, NJ: Rowman & Littlefield.

HARAWAY, D. (1988). Situated knowledges: The science question in feminism and the privilege of partial perspective. *Feminist Studies, 14*(3), 575–599.

JAGGAR, A. M. (1983). *Feminist politics and human nature.* Totowa, NJ: Rowman & Allanheld.

JONES, H. W. (1992). Assisted reproduction. *Clinical Obstetrics and Gynecology, 35*(4), 749–757.

KOSHY, M., & Burd, L. (1991). Management of pregnancy in sickle cell syndromes. *Hematology/Oncology Clinics of North America, 5*(3), 585–596.

LEMKE, A. (1992). Reproductive issues in adults with cystic fibrosis: Implications for genetic counseling. *Journal of Genetic Counseling, 1*(3), 211–218.

LIPPMAN, A. (1991). Prenatal genetic testing and screening: Constructing needs and reinforcing inequities. *American Journal of Law & Medicine, 17*(1–2), 15–50.

MAHOWALD, M. B. (1992). *Philosophy of woman: An anthology of classic and current concepts* (2nd ed.). Indianapolis: Hackett.

MAHOWALD, M. B. (1993). *Women and children in health care: An unequal majority.* New York: Oxford University Press.

NATOWICZ, M. R., Alper, J. K., & Alper, J. (1992). Genetic discrimination and the law. *American Journal of Human Genetics, 50,* 465–475.

NODDINGS, N. (1984). *Caring: A feminine approach to ethics and moral education.* Berkeley: University of California Press.

NOZICK, R. (1974). *Anarchy, state, and utopia.* New York: Basic Books.

NSIAH-JEFFERSON, L., & Hall, E. J. (1989). Reproductive technology: Perspectives and implications for low-income women and women of color. In K. S. Ratcliff, M. M. Ferree, G. O. Mellow, et al. (Eds.), *Healing technology: Feminist perspectives* (pp. 93–117). Ann Arbor: University of Michigan Press.

OKIN, S. M. (1989). *Justice, gender, and the family.* New York: Basic Books.

PEARCE, D. (1978). The feminization of poverty: Women, work and welfare. *Urban and Social Change Review, 11,* 28–36.

PENCARINHA, D. F., Bell, N. K., Edwards, J. G., & Best, R. G. (1992). Ethical issues in genetic counseling: A comparison of M.S. counselor and medical geneticist perspectives. *Journal of Genetic Counseling, 1*(1), 19–30.

RAWLS, J. (1971). *A theory of justice.* Cambridge, MA: Belknap Press of Harvard University Press.

REYNOLDS, B., Puck, M. H., & Robinson, A. (1974). Genetic counseling: An appraisal. *Clinical Genetics, 5,* 177–187.

RUDDICK, S. (1989). *Maternal thinking: Towards a politics of peace.* Boston: Beacon Press.

SHERWIN, S. (1992). *No longer patient: Feminist ethics and health care.* Philadelphia: Temple University Press.

TONG, R. (1989). *Feminist thought.* Boulder, CO: Westview Press.

TUCKER, R. (Ed.). (1972). *The Marx-Engels reader.* New York: Norton.

WARREN, V. L. (1989). Feminist directions in medical ethics. *Hypatia, 4,* 73–87.

WERTZ, D. C. (1993). Providers' gender and moral reasoning. *Fetal Diagnosis and Therapy, 8*(Suppl 1), 81–89.

WERTZ, D. C., & Fletcher, J. C. (1989). Moral reasoning among medical geneticists in eighteen nations. *Theoretical Medicine, 10,* 123–138.

WERTZ, D. C., & Fletcher, J. C. (1992). Ethical decision making in medical genetics: Women as patients and practitioners in eighteen nations. In K. S. Ratcliff, M. M. Ferree, G. O. Mellow, et al. (Eds.), *Healing technology: Feminist perspectives* (pp. 221–241). Ann Arbor: University of Michigan Press.

ZARE, N., Sorenson, J. R., & Heeren, T. (1984). Sex of provider as a variable in effective genetic counselling. *Social Science and Medicine, 19*(4), 671–675.

Reproductive Genetic Testing, Prevention, and the Ethics of Mothering

R U T H   F A D E N

Introduction

This chapter discusses whether pregnant women ought to obtain reproductive genetic testing.[1] This topic, and the particular way of framing the issues it represents, is, however, by no means the only or even the most important ethical consideration raised by reproductive genetic testing. Larger questions about the implications of advances in that area for the meaning of moral community are at least partially pushed to the background when the moral issues are particularized to the individual mother and child. Indeed, it could be argued that, from the standpoint of women, as well as that of persons with disabilities, it is on this wider social plane that the moral stakes are the highest.

Having said that, it is clear that reproductive genetic testing confronts each of us as individuals, as pregnant woman or other, with important ethical questions. From the perspective of the morality of personal action, at least four kinds of questions need addressing:

1. Should pregnant women seek reproductive genetic testing?

2. Should pregnant women accept offers of reproductive genetic testing?

3. Should pregnant women seek or accept therapeutic interventions suggested by genetic testing?

4. What, in the absence of therapy, should pregnant women do when a fetus is identified as having a "problem"?

Two Approaches

Consider the following proposition. Pregnant women ought to take reasonable steps to use genetic technology to prevent or reduce illness or disability in their prospective children (fetuses that pregnant women are carrying to term). A defense of this proposition can be constructed in numerous ways, including both a traditional analysis from principle and an analysis from an ethic of care (an ethic of care being one of several contemporary challenges to traditional moral theory with ties to feminism and feminist moral psychology [Blustein, 1991; Carse, 1991; Sherwin, 1992]).

In an analysis from principle, the central task is determining whether there exists a maternal duty to employ genetic interventions, where duty is understood as a fixed obligation grounded in either a single moral principle or some combination of moral principles. The most promising candidates for grounding a maternal duty to employ genetic interventions are the principles of nonmaleficence and beneficence.

The principle of nonmaleficence holds that one ought not inflict harm or evil upon others. The implications of this powerful but general moral injunction for parental duties toward genetic testing are not, however, straightforward. Jeffrey Kahn has undertaken the most exhaustive analysis of this topic to date. As Kahn points out, it is by no means clear whether the passing on of a "bad gene" constitutes the inflicting of a harm, nor is it clear in what sense persons can be harmed by their genes, or what act (such as conception, failing to terminate the pregnancy, or failing to interfere with the pregnancy) is the particular act that harms.

By contrast to the complexities of relating maternal duties to nonmaleficence, an analysis from the principle of beneficence

has considerable intuitive appeal. Although the principle of beneficence is also concerned about harm—its removal or prevention—the principle primarily considers duties in terms of con-
ferring benefits or seeking the best interests of others. Thus, for
genetic testing to fall under the scope of the beneficence principle, thorny conceptual problems about the nature of harm and
harming need not be resolved. All that is required is an assumption that the interests of offspring would best be served, that
offspring would be better off, if their mothers were to employ
(at least some) genetic interventions.

The problem with applying the principle of beneficence is the
principle's indeterminacy, its disputed moral standing with respect to the imposition of strict moral duties. There is virtually
no dispute that individuals have strong (negative) obligations to
refrain from harming others. By contrast, there is considerable
disagreement about whether, under what conditions, and to
what extent individuals have positive obligations to benefit others. The central problem is how to fix such duties of beneficence. A typical maneuver is to move from an analysis of general duties of beneficence to an analysis of duties specific to
particular roles. That is, even if we cannot agree about the existence of general moral obligations to benefit others, surely
certain roles carry with them very fixed and specific duties to
benefit others. A paradigmatic such role is that of mother. Assuming we can accept that mothers have strict duties of beneficence toward their children, an application to the context of reproductive genetic testing requires evidence that the use of at
least some such testing falls within those duties. For this claim
to be sustained, it is necessary to establish that maternal duties
of beneficence apply to prospective children as well as children
already born, and that the use of (at least some) genetic interventions are in the best interests of those prospective children.

The question of whether pregnant women ought to take reasonable steps to use genetic technology to prevent or reduce
illness or disability in their prospective children can also be ap-
proached from the perspective of an ethic of care. Rather than
working from a structure of moral principles, the focus of a
care-based ethic is on the moral nature of relationships and on a
way of thinking about the moral life that has as its foundational

moral categories not rights and duties, but commitment, empathy, compassion, caring, and love. Here again, the paradigmatic context is the family and, especially, the parent-child relationship. It has been argued, I think correctly, that the parent-child relationship is better analyzed in terms of moral categories like caring, compassion, and love than by a language of impersonal, objective rights and duties (Blustein, 1989). Indeed, it seems incontrovertible that caring and love rest in the essence of parenting, that what it means to be a parent, above else, is to care for and seek the welfare of one's child. Ensuring or enhancing the health and functioning of one's child is surely part of what it means to care for one's child. Thus, insofar as reproductive genetic testing and related interventions can contribute to the (prospective) child's welfare, seeking such interventions would fall within the moral territory of parenting.

There are many ambiguities, many unanalyzed nuances in this sketchy presentation, both with respect to an analysis from principle or from an ethic of care. One common point worthy of emphasis, however, is that neither approach relies on any argument that is unique to genetics or to reproduction. In both cases, the appeal is grounded in a general understanding that mothers are supposed to seek and protect the health of their children—including taking reasonable steps to prevent illness or disability—and that, at least in theory, genetic testing can contribute to that end. What is left open in this sketchy treatment is the specific meaning of such critical terms as prevention and "reasonable steps." Although a careful analysis of these complex concepts is beyond the scope of this chapter, a few comments are in order.

Prevention

Despite prevention's venerable history in medicine, and especially in public health where the term has been parsed in numerous ways, no rigorous analysis exists of what it means to prevent illness or disability (as opposed, for example, to treatment or rehabilitation). Particularly with respect to genetics, the boundaries of the concept of prevention remain largely unchartered. Perhaps the most troubling question is whether or in

what sense the term prevention can be applied to eugenic policies and practices. For example, when a program of maternal
serum alpha-fetoprotein screening results in the abortion of ten
fetuses identified as having neural tube defects, is this conceptually or morally analogous to a hypertension screening program's resulting in the averting of ten cases of untreated malig-
nant hypertension?

From a moral perspective, the answer to this question is an
emphatic No. Eliminating an incident of disease or disability by
"preventing" the person who would have that disease or disability from being born is not an instance of prevention—not in
the sense in which it is ordinarily meant and not as the term
ought to be used. As has been argued elsewhere, treating the
prevention of the birth of children who would have an illness or
disability as morally equivalent to preventing illness or disability in persons already living involves a morally unacceptable
view of the worth of such persons (Asch, 1989; Faden, Geller,
& Powers, 1991). It suggests that the lives of some persons with
a disability or illness are not worth living, that such persons are
to be understood only as social or economic drains and never as
sources of either independent value or enrichment for the lives
of others.

From the perspective of the morality of mothering, it similarly can be argued that preventing illness or disability in children already living is morally different from preventing the
birth of a child who would have an illness or disability. Maternal commitments to care for one's children, to seek their interests, and to spare them disease and disability thus do not extend
to or encompass preventing the birth of such children (whether
by selective abortion, selective conception, or remaining childless). To hold otherwise, one must be able to argue that it is in
the child's interests not to be born, that life with the disease or
disability is so poor and aversive that it is a life not worth living
or a life worse than no life at all.[2]

Can this condition ever be satisfied? According to some commentators the answer to this question is no, if only because the
comparing of any state of existence with nonexistence is meta-
physically or logically impossible (Tedeschi, 1966). Still others
have argued that such a comparison is possible and that non-

existence may indeed be preferable when, for example, it would be rational to prefer death to existence or when all and every interest in life is doomed from the outset (Feinberg, 1986; Parfit, 1986).

It is arguably the case that very few genetic disorders meet such criteria. (Lesch–Nyhan syndrome, a devastating genetic disease that results in mental retardation, self-mutilation, and renal failure, may be one such instance.) It follows that, allowing for the rare exception, there is no requirement *in mothering* to seek or accept reproductive genetic testing if the only actions facilitated by such testing are abortion, selective conception, or remaining childless. Implicit in this position is a rejection of abortion as, in any sense, a therapy for the fetus. Moreover, as a pragmatic matter, this means that today, given the paucity of effective, available therapies, women striving to be good mothers should not feel under any obligation to accept reproductive genetic testing out of a sense of commitment to or compassion for their prospective children.

It does not follow from this position, however, that seeking reproductive genetic testing for purposes of selective abortion is necessarily morally wrong. The claim is only that, from the perspective of the moral context of mothering a prospective child, no moral requirement to have reproductive genetic testing exists in the absence of effective therapy for that child. This said, it must be recognized that commitments to other family members or to oneself can provide reasons to elect genetic testing and selective abortion and that those reasons may be morally or prudentially compelling.

Reasonable Steps

Assuming an effective therapy for the prospective child is available, what can pregnant women reasonably be expected to endure in the way of personal hardship, loss of liberty, or risk of harm in order to secure that therapy? The answer to this question is in many respects more difficult than are those to questions about prevention and genetic intervention. Although duties of beneficence may seem more clearly applicable to the maternal role than to other contexts, the nature and boundaries of maternal duties of beneficence are by no means understood. Among feminist scholars and other proponents of an ethics of care, there is a growing literature on the meaning of mothering and the moral dimensions of familial bonds.[3] Still, many questions remain unanswered. Perhaps most fundamentally, how are we to understand commitment, self-effacement, and ultimately love in the context of parenting when what is considered by some to be heroic self-sacrifice on the part of a mother is considered by others to be nothing more than a standard instance of good mothering?

It is at this juncture that gender differences potentially loom large. At least for the foreseeable future, it is likely that many genetic interventions of benefit to prospective children will have to be delivered through the bodies of their pregnant mothers. How does bodily integrity and personal physical risk alter the dynamic, in moral terms, of the mother-child or parent-child relationship? My own view is that, if the stakes for the child are high enough, parents—both mothers and fathers—ought to accept some level of pain and physical risk to aid their child. If, for example, a father refused to be a kidney donor for his child when his kidney was clearly the child's best chance for survival then, barring mitigating circumstances, that father would be morally beneath contempt. Similarly, if fetal surgery could spare a prospective child severe disability or illness, then (again, barring mitigating circumstances) a pregnant woman's refusal of the surgery would be morally reprehensible.

Having said that, it should be emphasized that whether and to what extent mothers should, in a particular context, take actions that benefit their children is a separate inquiry from whether and to what extent state or professional action should encourage or compel pregnant women to behave accordingly. That is, from the finding that a woman would be morally wrong in refusing a genetic intervention that would significantly benefit her prospective child, it does not follow that the state would be right in compelling that pregnant woman to have the intervention, or that a health professional would be right in manipulating the woman into accepting the intervention. Such questions of public policy must take into account considerations external to the maternal-child relationship. The oppressive history of restrictions on the medical decisions of women, especially pregnant women, and the destructive effects on women of social values and policies that view us dominantly as vessels for protecting the unborn loom large in any discussion of coercive or manipulative public policies. Indeed, it is at the level of public policy, and not personal morality, that historical and social differences between women and men may in the end be the most morally relevant.

Conclusion

Although a full account of the moral dimensions of mothering has yet to be developed, any plausible analysis would likely support the position that pregnant women ought to use reproductive genetic technology if the technology results in interventions that could prevent or reduce significant illness or disability in the child after birth. The moral justification for using such technology in the absence of therapy for the child must rest on considerations external to the relationship of the mother to the prospective child—including, for example, commitments to existing children, other family members, or oneself. In both private and public discourse, it is important that we be honest about our reasons for considering and justifying reproductive genetic testing. When a mother of normal intelligence prevents the birth of a child with Down syndrome, or when a deaf mother prevents the birth of a hearing child, they may be legitimately furthering their own interests or those of others in their family or community. They cannot plausibly claim their action is in the best interest of the child who as a consequence will never be born.

NOTES

1. Much of this analysis applies as well to prospective fathers who, for example, may be called upon to undergo carrier testing in a reproductive context.
2. Both Steinbock (1992) and Arras (1990) have developed arguments defending less stringent criteria for determining when it is in the interests of a child (who would be born) to terminate a pregnancy.
3. See Held (1987), Okin (1989), Rothman (1989), Ruddick (1992), Sommers (1987), Treblicot (1983), and Whitbeck (1986).

BIBLIOGRAPHY

ARRAS, J. (1990). AIDS and reproductive decisions: Having children in fear and trembling. *Milbank Memorial Quarterly, 68,* 353–382.

ASCH, A. (1989). Reproductive technology and disability. In S. Cohen & N. Taub (Eds.), *Reproductive Laws for the 1990's* (pp. 69–107). Clifton, NJ: Humana Press.

BLUSTEIN, J. (1989). The rights approach and the intimacy approach. *Mount Sinai Journal of Medicine, 56,* 164–167.

BLUSTEIN, J. (1991). *Care and commitment.* New York: Oxford University Press.

CARSE, A. L. (1991). The "voice" of care. *The Journal of Medicine and Philosophy, 16,* 5–28.

FADEN, R. R., Geller, G., & Powers, M. (1991). *AIDS, women and the next generation.* New York: Oxford University Press.

FEINBERG, J. (1986). Wrongful life and the counterfactual element in harming. *Social Philosophy and Policy, 4,* 145–178.

HELD, V. (1987). Feminism and moral theory. In E. F. Kittay & D. T. Meyers (Eds.), *Women and moral theory* (pp. 11–128). Totowa, NJ: Rowman & Littlefield.

KAHN, J. (1989). The principle of nonmaleficence and the problems of reproductive decision making (doctoral dissertation). Georgetown University Department of Philosophy.

OKIN, S. K. (1989). *Justice, gender, and the family.* New York: Basic Books.

PARFIT, D. (1986). *Reasons and persons.* Oxford: Oxford University Press.

ROTHMAN, B. K. (1989). *Recreating motherhood: Ideology and technology in a patriarchal society.* New York: Norton.

RUDDICK, S. (1992). From maternal thinking to peace politics. In E. B. Cole & S. Coultrap-Mcquin (Eds.), *Explorations in feminist ethics* (pp. 141–155). Bloomington: Indiana University Press.

SHERWIN, S. (1992). *No longer patient: Feminist ethics and health care.* Philadelphia: Temple University Press.

SOMMERS, C. H. (1987). Filial morality. In E. F. Kittay & D. T. Meyers (Eds.), *Women and moral theory* (pp. 69–84). Totowa, NJ: Rowman & Littlefield.

STEINBOCK, B. (1992). *The moral and legal status of embryos and fetuses.* New York: Oxford University Press.

TEDESCHI, G. (1966). On tort liability for wrongful life. *Israeli Law Review, 1,* 513–538.

TREBLICOT, J. (Ed.). (1983). *Mothering: Essays in feminist theory*. Totowa, NJ: Rowman & Allanheld.

WHITBECK, C. (1986). The moral dimensions of regarding women as people. In W. B. Bondesman, H. T. Engelhardt, S. F. Spicker, & D. Winship (Eds.), *Abortion and the status of the fetus*. Dordrecht: Reidel.

6 Ethics and Reproductive Genetic Testing:

The Need to Understand the Parent-Child Relationship

PATRICIA A. KING

Reproductive genetic testing raises complex and perplexing ethical issues. Why is this so? In significant part, the reason is that the dilemmas posed by reproductive genetic testing implicate the parent-child relationship. Ethics and law lack an adequate theoretical basis for understanding the structure and functioning of the family—especially the parent-child relationship. Therefore, those who wish to resolve ethical issues in reproductive genetic testing are seriously hindered.

It is particularly difficult to conceptualize the duties and obligations that should revolve around the parent-child relationship. The two parties are not strangers; thus, it would be inappropriate to assume that they will be motivated primarily by self-interest. Conceptualizing this relationship is further complicated by the fact that the parties involved are not of equivalent status: the fetus is always dependent and vulnerable.

The parent-child relationship is linked to an understanding of women's biological and social roles. Only women gestate. In addition, childrearing has been and continues to be the overwhelming responsibility of women. Although men are biological parents and are responsible for the care of children, the parenting role is not culturally understood to be a defining one for them.

The most perplexing aspects of the parent-child relationship involve the decision of whether, and under what conditions, a

98

pregnancy should be initiated, and if so, what the appropriate treatment of the fetus should be. These issues go to the heart of the ethical and policy-making questions raised by reproductive genetic testing. Moreover, to a large degree it has been the advances in genetic and reproductive technologies that have highlighted the lack of a sufficient theoretical account of the parent-child relationship. The need for an adequate analytical framework will assume even greater urgency as current efforts to map and sequence the human genome progress.

Genetic and reproductive technologies have increased the power of individuals (and couples) to decide whether to procreate and whether to control the size, timing, and desirable characteristics of offspring. Not only have those advances opened up new possibilities for individual reproductive choice, they have also provided governments and private institutions with more efficient methods of coercing reproductive choices. For example, both governments and private institutions can refuse to pay medical costs incurred by a child who was prenatally diagnosed as having a genetic disease but not aborted.

To make matters more complex, increased options for individuals, private institutions, and the state have become available at the same time that the family itself is undergoing profound change. The elevated status of women and children within the traditional family is changing the roles of family members and the nature of interactions among them, while the growth of single-parent families is a stark reminder of the reality that women and children increasingly live in nontraditional environments.

In short, guidance for private and public policy decisions in reproductive genetic testing is urgently needed, yet difficult to provide. Below I will identify the areas implicated by the parent-child relationship that I believe are most in need of attention if we are to make progress in resolving the dilemmas posed by reproductive genetics.

The critical issue at hand is the need for an understanding of the parent-child relationship, including the period of pregnancy, that is grounded in the experiences of parents in their relationships with offspring. I agree with those who argue that a "language shift" is needed. A language shift is undeniably linked with the need for a different conceptual framework. Terms and concepts such as choice, autonomy, rights, and non-interference, do not capture my own experiential understanding of pregnancy or of parenting after birth, nor do they capture what I can remember of my experiences as a child.

These terms and concepts seem especially problematic in the context of my experience of pregnancy. Pregnancy is typically described from the perspective of either the woman and her rights, or the fetus and its rights. Such descriptions tend to oversimplify matters. In my experience, a woman who wants to have a child sees herself as involved in a relationship with the fetus—a relationship that is not adversarial or antagonistic. The fetus is both a part of a woman's body and a separate, distinct entity that may suffer injury not suffered by the woman. A woman's experience of pregnancy is thus complex, informed with multiple meanings, not fully captured by language that emphasizes separateness and rights.

Moreover, a woman does not exist with her fetus or child in isolation; she may have relationships with other children, a spouse, family members, or significant others. Decisions that she makes with respect to any one of those relationships must take into account her involvement with all of the others. There needs to be a way to include the contextual nature of a woman's decision-making. I am not sure what the language or concepts should be—obligation, duty, responsibility, care, love, compassion?—but there is a clear need to move away from the existing language and its conceptual implications. In short, we need a different analytical approach that focuses on relationships where one party is dependent and vulnerable.

Whatever form a revised framework takes, it should contain a broad and inclusive understanding of who a parent is and what it means to parent—again, an understanding anchored in the experiences of parenting. An ongoing problem has been that reproduction has primarily been associated with women. Yet there is no reason why male responsibilities should not also be addressed. One of the implications of using terms such as responsibility, obligation, and care is that they are not limited in their applicability to women. These terms serve as reminders that men are also parents. From my perspective as parent, wife, and former child, involving men in parenting responsibilities serves only to benefit us all.

What must parenting entail? Often parenting is discussed as though it requires total sacrifice of the parents' interests. While many parents may indeed strive for sainthood, parenting cannot require such complete sacrifice in the name of the best interests of the child any more than it permits utterly self-interested behavior. A balance needs to be struck. Too much self-interest is detrimental to children. However, requiring total sacrifice of parental interests would be burdensome, and persons would choose other ways of occupying their time. Moreover, parents must sometimes consider the needs of others. Parenting a child does not exist in isolation from the needs of other children, dependent persons, or even of spouses and friends.

A better understanding of what it means to parent raises the possibility that acting responsibly may encompass a decision not to parent. This is not an idea that has received sufficient attention; it arises quite naturally, however, in the context of genetics and prenatal diagnosis of disease. Let me hasten to add that I absolutely agree with the view expressed by several authors that the decision to terminate a pregnancy after prenatal diagnosis of a genetic disease cannot be justified as being in the fetus's best interests. A decision to terminate a pregnancy might nonetheless be a responsible decision in view of the needs and life circumstances of the pregnant woman and those affected by her decisions. I was recently told the story of one pregnant woman with an existing child who recounted that she really didn't agree with abortion, but believed she must have one because she felt she should focus on the needs of the child she already had. A new child would mean that her existing child would not receive all of the attention it needed. The view expressed by that woman may be difficult for some to understand, but given certain circumstances, it makes a great deal of sense to me.

Finally, in thinking about what parenting might entail, we need to keep in mind that women come from many cultures, ethnic groups, and economic classes. Our ethics therefore should be contextual not abstract in nature. It must take into account the infinite varieties of family life and relationships. My family law students are given to saying, "a reasonable mother would . . ." They are reassured by the notion that there can be some high degree of objectivity in describing the role of parents. I prefer to emphasize what a reasonable parent would do *under the circumstances*—an emphasis that draws attention to the problem of generalization. I also stress the difficulty of outsiders' truly being able to appreciate all of the circumstances in others' lives.

Shifting to different paradigms, however, is not risk-free. We live in a society that wants to make ethical requirements legal ones—to compel behavior to conform to objective norms. Thus, prevailing norms of parental responsibility become forces that shape when, how, and with whom the state should intervene. For example, a "strong" view of parental obligation has often implied that the state should help only when parental resources are exhausted or otherwise unavailable. When the state in its role as provider of last resort supplies resources, moreover, it does so only to help the weak, vulnerable, or dependent *individual* as opposed to the family unit or the parent. A "strong" view of family obligation may also be used to justify punishment of family members who are perceived as not meeting parental obligations. As a consequence, many fear, with good cause, that a focus on parental obligation rather than on rights is an invitation to greater interference by the state into the lives of individual parents than is desirable.

We must not forget that technological innovations have the potential to vastly expand parental options about reproduction and the characteristics of offspring. Economic, social, and demographic changes have the potential to continue to alter our traditional understanding of the family, its structure, and inherent responsibilities. Significant changes in social expectations about parenting may result. This is particularly a problem in genetics. The President's Commission in 1983 warned of this possibility in the context of prenatal therapy. It stated:

> If the capacity to perform prenatal therapy expands, significant changes are likely to occur in social expectations about parental and societal obligations to the unborn. . . .
> One aspect of this change would be more demanding so-

cial expectations of parents in promoting the welfare of the fetus. So although the developments in prenatal therapy increase the range of technically feasible options, social pressures may severely limit parents' freedom to refrain from choosing certain options.[1]

In the context of reproductive genetic testing, there could be increased pressure to reduce the degree of choice permitted in these decisions, in the interest of the collective goal to reduce the incidence of genetic disease.

Related is the concern that state involvement in individual reproductive decision-making will not fall equally across the population. The vulnerable—women, minorities, and the poor—will bear the greatest burdens, as historical evidence corroborates. Women, in particular, fear that a conceptual framework focusing on responsibility, obligation, and care too closely resembles earlier definitions of women's roles that served to oppress and disadvantage women in relation to men.

Those risks are real, and current frameworks have proven inadequate. Risks can be ameliorated, however, by taking into account several factors: First, the ability to protect bodily integrity—especially the body's reproductive functions—is critical to self-identity and should not lightly be ignored. Second, while legal regulation of the parent-child relationship might be appropriate in some situations, it is difficult, if not impossible, for law to require all of the endless care and kindnesses toward others that we associate with intimate, and sometimes dependent, relationships. Third, historically, ethics and law have permitted a broad range of parenting behaviors. We should move away from this perspective only with the greatest of caution. Finally, and perhaps of the greatest importance, many parents are willing to act in the interests of their children, but may not have the training, resources, knowledge, skills, or fortitude to act without support from others (including the state) to carry out their responsibilities.

A revised framework for understanding the parent-child relationship must therefore include a basis for protecting the privacy traditionally associated with parental decision-making without unduly exposing vulnerable persons to harm. At the same time, this framework must recognize that no families are alike and that some require affirmative assistance rather than punishment in order to meet their own expectations and the expectations of society as a whole.

NOTES

1. President's Commission for the Study of Ethical Problems in Medicine and Biomedical and Behavioral Research, Report on Screening and Counseling for Genetic Conditions, 1983, p. 54, note 14.

7

"The Good Mother":

The Limits of Reproductive
Accountability and Genetic Choice

R. ALTA CHARO AND
KAREN H. ROTHENBERG

Bree Walker Lampley has discovered the meaning of the feminist truism that the personal *is* the political. A Southern Californian television news anchor, with a genetic condition that causes her to suffer missing or fused toes and fingers, Bree Walker Lampley became the subject of public discussion about whether it was appropriate to conceive a child who faced a 50–50 chance of inheriting the same condition. In a breathtaking display of insensitivity, a local radio talk show host held a two-hour call-in discussion of Walker Lampley's decision on the issue. At the time, Walker Lampley was seven months pregnant.

Underlying the controversy surrounding the talk show, and indeed the amorphous fears surrounding the Human Genome Project, is the perpetual question of accountability. Should women be held accountable for the size, health, and demographic makeup of future generations? The question is asked in terms of women's accountability because it is they who conceive, gestate, and give birth to these generations. Governments have often looked to women's reproductive decisions as the mediating mechanism for enforcing a social policy on population size and structure. In many ways, fertile women are viewed as having the "last clear chance" (in the jargon of tort law) to perpetuate or stifle a genetic trait. The question is, does the public have a legitimate interest in that choice? If so, are women therefore accountable to the public for the choices they make? Are they accountable to their families and to the children with genetic disorders they bring into the world?

The question is more than hypothetical. A 1990 general population survey revealed that 39% feel that "every woman who is pregnant should be tested to determine if the baby has genetic defects," and 22% believe that, regardless of what they would want for themselves, "a woman should have an abortion if the baby has a serious genetic defect" (Singer, 1991). Nearly 10% stated they believe that poor women should be required to abort fetuses with genetic disorders rather than be allowed to turn to government assistance for the child's rearing and health care. With regard to specific disorders, surveys reveal that 95% of women would choose abortion following prenatal diagnosis of severe mental retardation, and 60% for moderate mental retardation, blindness, or paraplegia (Benn et al., 1985; Faden et al., 1987; Golbus et al., 1979).

On the other hand, parents of children with a genetic disorder such as cystic fibrosis are more tolerant. They tend to support both the choice to have more children with genetic disorders and the choice to terminate pregnancy upon request. For example, a substantial majority support the right to legal abortion in the first trimester following diagnosis of any of the aforementioned disorders, and 58% would themselves have an abortion in the face of a fetus with severe mental retardation. On the other hand, only 40% would themselves abort a fetus with a disorder leading to death before age five; 35%, a fetus predicted to develop moderate mental retardation; 20%, a fetus affected with cystic fibrosis; and 17%, a fetus predicted to develop a severe, incurable disease with onset at age forty (Wertz et al., 1991). This disparity between tolerating and choosing abortion among those with personal experience relating to a child born with a genetic disorder highlights the intensely personal nature of these decisions, and the inability of those most closely associated with such circumstances to agree upon bright-lined rules concerning responsible reproductive behavior.

This chapter first examines the question of personal accountability to one's family or children for reproductive decisions. It concludes that while arguments can be made for moral accountability, legal accountability is inappropriate for the following reasons: First, conundrums concerning causation and calculation of damages make legal remedies difficult to fashion. Second, legal accountability adds little to the already significant emotional and financial forces constraining reproductive choice in the face of probable genetic disorder. Finally, legal accountability is premised on the notion that there are indeed objective standards measuring those lives that are worth living and those that are not, an assertion we reject. The chapter then shifts to the question of whether to hold women publicly accountable to the community for their reproductive decisions. Following an analysis of the political and ethical underpinnings of individual rights and community interests, we conclude that justifications to manipulate women's reproductive decisions are fatally flawed.

Personal Accountability for Having a Child with Genetic Disorders

A woman's decision to conceive, abort, or bear a child with genetic disorders may be subject to questions of personal, as well as communal, accountability. To argue for such a moral or legal accountability requires that one view the decision to use or forego genetic testing as a voluntary and informed choice that is causally related to some subsequent harm. Those assumptions, however, are not well founded.

Nondirective counseling and the informed consent process are based on our assumption that patient choice is a given. Proponents of reproductive genetic testing argue that with more genetic information there will be more choice. In fact, the availability of reproductive genetic testing assumes several levels of choice: whether to have a test, what to learn from the test, whether to live with uncertainty about its results, and whether to carry to term. But choice is not that simple. From the preconception stage forward, choice free of situational coercion may be an illusion. As an example, for those women who have little or no access to prenatal care, genetic services are not available. It is therefore inappropriate to speak of their "choice" to forego genetically indicated abortion in the context of assigning moral or legal blame.

This lack of choice can be illustrated by an examination of available genetic screening services. Federal funds are available for limited screening, but not for the abortion that some women would choose in the light of certain results (Clayton, 1993; NARAL, 1992). The majority of states place similar limitations on the use of public funds (NARAL, 1992). And the *Webster v. Reproductive Health Services*[1] decision upheld the constitutionality of prohibiting the use of not only public funds, but also public facilities or public personnel, for abortion services. Nor is adequate funding available at the state or federal level to ensure even minimal health care for every child brought to term despite prenatal diagnoses of genetic disorder. Thus, even if screening is available, financial considerations will constrain the resulting "choices" concerning procreation to the point that moral and legal responsibility for the outcome may be dubious.

Given those limitations, how can impoverished women be held personally accountable for reproductive decisions following genetic counseling? And if such parental responsibility could be assigned, should it not be shared by both parents, even if one parent—the mother—has a constitutionally protected veto power over decisions concerning abortion?

In an ideal world, carrier screening prior to pregnancy would be a joint responsibility of the couple. Obtaining information about probabilities of genetic risk may help to clarify decision-making about reproduction, and this is a shared responsibility. However, once the decision is made to conceive and the egg has been fertilized, the responsibility shifts exclusively to the woman. This is so regardless of whether she is the carrier of the risky genetic link. The decision to conceive, often tied to the need for genetic connection by both parents, shifts all responsibility related with genetic testing to the mother: she is the sole subject of testing. In this context, do her husband's or partner's desires make her choice less than fully voluntary? If so, then moral accountability and legal concepts of proximate cause are obscured.

A further compromise of autonomous decision-making arises from the problems involved in developing standards of prenatal care practice. Providers, who set the standard of care, have a choice not to provide such testing. But some providers may feel compelled to encourage women to choose genetic testing, both out of concern for the outcome of the birth and for fear of legal liability (U.S. Congress, 1992). Ironically, the more the profession encourages genetic testing and increases consumer expectations, the more it will be trapped into providing the services due to the perceived threat of medical malpractice litigation. Nonetheless, the profession has the power and the responsibility to question risks and benefits of genetic testing in the broader context of comprehensive pregnancy care. One example might be to attempt to educate the public as to how rarely genetic abnormalities significantly impair a baby's health.

Professional conflict of interest can also compromise genetic counseling. The counseling session is often scheduled just prior to the genetic testing itself so that the woman may sign a consent form. There could instead be a greater interval recommended between counseling and testing procedures, allowing the woman to consider fully all of the relevant issues. Genetic counselors should not feel that they have failed themselves or their employers if a woman chooses not to be tested, nor should a woman's decision to forego testing have financial consequences for the counselors or their employers.

In addition, genetic counseling should make clear what options a woman will have after receiving test results. Obviously, there has been increasing concern that as both the use and scope of genetic testing are expanding, the constitutional right to choose to terminate a pregnancy is contracting. While protecting previability abortion decisions from many state restrictions, recent Supreme Court decisions still tolerate extreme limits on postviability abortion—even for genetic indications—and permit mandatory counseling throughout the pregnancy period as a condition of obtaining abortion services. This makes it likely that each state will set its own rules for categorizing those conditions that justify postviability abortion. Some states will allow such abortions for "fetal defect," congenital anomalies and the like, but as reproductive testing increases, legislation will have to refine and adjust those definitions. For example, some genetic aberrations do not cause significant disorder of physical health, but can create cosmetic problems that are likely to cause disorder of mental health due to societal reactions to the child's appearance. Whether they will constitute a "defect" poses a problem of enormous emotional and political dimensions.

The Supreme Court's decision in *Planned Parenthood of Pennsylvania v. Casey*[2] also sheds light on the permissible range of State restrictions on abortion that may affect the use of genetic services. The Supreme Court held that mandatory counseling requirements are permissible expressions of state interest in the protection of fetal life and in preference for childbirth over abortion, so long as they do not become an undue burden on a woman's right to obtain previability abortions, which the court did reaffirm as an aspect of protected personal liberty. Mandatory counseling introduces the opinions of the physician, the genetic counselor, and, in the case of counseling directives written by the state, the opinions of the state legislature and regulators as well. The *Casey* decision specifically upholds the constitutionality of state measures designed to express a state preference for childbirth over abortion. This includes any form of counseling that presents objectively accurate information, even if it is an unbalanced presentation, so long as the counseling does not amount to an "undue burden." The politics of the disability rights movement and the anti-abortion movement could well result in a rash of mandatory counseling provisions designed to discourage couples from using prenatal diagnosis for selective termination of pregnancy. Twenty-five states already have mandatory counseling legislation (NARAL, 1992).

As noted above, such provisions might also incorporate state attempts to define "genetic defect" in a way that manipulates parental responses to test results. States as diverse as Delaware and Texas have attempted in the past to limit abortions to cases of "severe" or "grave" malformations or defects (Clayton, 1993). Under *Casey*, it would appear states may still attempt to mandate counseling that characterizes some genetic conditions as minor and others as severe. A key question in such statutes is the definition of "severe defect." First, a number of test results from genetic screening can be ambiguous. Some forms of mosaicism or triploidy, for example, can be difficult to evaluate. Even in easily identified disorders, such as cystic fibrosis, the expression of the disease can be highly variable, and the state of the art in treatment is still rapidly evolving. Whether such a condition represents a "severe defect" is a matter of interpretation.

Even more important in such a scenario is the identity of the person making the interpretation of "minor" versus "severe." In many cases this will be the physician, who will need to certify that the statutory counseling requirements were met before an abortion was performed. But the varying attitude toward abortion and disability among physicians will certainly make this judgment itself highly variable, even within a community, let alone among jurisdictions.

Furthermore, the *Rust v. Sullivan*[3] decision upheld an interpretation of Title X regulations that prevents federally funded clinics from providing any sort of abortion counseling, except in cases of extreme medical need. Genetic abnormalities of the fetus would not provide an exception. Even following the repeal of the federal gag rule under the Clinton-Gore administration (APN, 1993), state legislation may continue to present such barriers. Louisiana, Missouri, and North Dakota, for example, have gag rules that mimic the federal restrictions on abortion counseling in publicly financed facilities (NARAL, 1992).

In addition to such financial and informational barriers, the profession itself often limits choice by abandoning the care of the pregnant woman midstream. The medical profession should ensure that providers making referrals for genetic testing or providing the genetic testing services also provide abortion services. The medical profession needs to better coordinate such services for the woman. At the same time that training in genetic testing is expanding, training in abortion services among residency programs is decreasing. At present, only 15% of the obstetrics-gynecology residents are trained in abortion procedures (O. Nordberg, personal communication, October 1992). Without such continuity, providers are in fact limiting choice for women.

Finally, lack of health insurance or information about disability services may also make some women feel they have no choice but to abort. Such women may worry that failure to abort will waive future support for the child born with disabilities. This fear may be real, as anecdotal reports continue to circulate (albeit rarely) of insurance companies and HMOs threatening not to cover expenses for children born by choice with genetic disorders (U.S. Congress, 1992).

Even if a woman's decision regarding procreation is made free of the economic and psychological constraints described above, it is difficult to argue that her decision "caused" any harm. The questions raised by wrongful birth and wrongful life actions may help illustrate the point.

A wrongful birth action assumes that by the provider's failure to disclose information about genetic testing or to provide the correct test result, the provider caused a harm that requires compensation to the parents of a child born with a genetic disorder.[4] The harm inflicted in this case is not that the child was born with a genetic disorder. Rather, the harm is the parents' deprivation of their right to know about a testable genetic condition and to then choose whether to terminate the pregnancy.

On the other hand, most courts have been unwilling to recognize a wrongful life action brought by a child against a provider for the same negligent conduct. In wrongful life, the child asserts it would have been better never to have been born than to live with such a severe disorder. Here, the provider has not actively harmed the child; that harm was caused by the accident of genetic disorder. The provider's action with respect to the child was at most a failure to "rescue" the child from a life of disorder by giving the parents timely information that would have led to an abortion. But the majority of courts are uncomfortable with any decision that hints that nonexistence might be preferable to a life with disability, and thus implicitly reject the notion that there is a duty to the child to rescue the child from such a life. Where there is no duty, there can be no cause of action or legal accountability.

These same considerations militate against legitimizing wrongful life actions by children against their parents. Unless one can find a duty to rescue a child from a life with unavoidable genetic disorders, one cannot hold the parent accountable for such a birth, even if the parent had sufficient options that the decision is correctly characterized as a "choice." Certainly, the goals of tort law are not served by holding mothers (as opposed to providers) accountable to children for the decision to give them life. Even assuming that there is a legitimate public purpose in reducing the number of children born with significant genetic disorders, maternal liability is pointless. A woman who faces the prospect of rearing a child with significant physical problems due to a genetic anomaly already has as much cautionary information as she needs. Adding the prospect of financial liability will add little to the already inherent deterring factors.

Nor does making a mother compensate her child for the pain incurred by life with genetic disorders serve as more than a dollar-shifting mechanism, moving money from the parent to the child. As parents already owe their children a duty of adequate support, it adds little to the child's opportunities for medical care. While lodging the suit against the parents' insurers may offer the prospect of additional dollars flowing into the family, it hardly seems reasonable to argue that the opportunity for fraudulent use of the insurance system should be offered to a suffering child. This is especially true in the light of the real prospect, on much more solid conceptual grounds, of recovery against those medical professionals (and their insurers) who failed to give the information necessary to allow parents to avoid such a birth.

Finally, there is little "justice" in holding women liable for choosing to give birth to afflicted children. In the tort system it is considered just when those who impose nonreciprocal risks upon others are required to pay for the privilege via compensation to the victim. But choosing to rear a child with disorders is not the imposition of a nonreciprocal risk: the risk is mutual. The parent risks deep regret at having taken on such a draining and difficult task. The child risks deep regret at having been given the opportunity to decide whether this sort of life is better than nonexistence. Admittedly, only one party can be in a position to make the choice; the as-yet unconceived child cannot have had any say. But absent an outright eugenic ban on having children while knowing they will be genetically disabled, the fact of the matter is that someone must choose; and that person can only be the parent. Indeed, who better than Bree Walker Lampley, herself affected by a genetic disorder, to balance the quality of her child's life against the task of raising such a child?

Who better than Bree Walker Lampley who has herself experienced the kinds of challenges her child will face?

Public Accountability and the Manipulation of Reproductive Decisions

Women are often subjected to communal, as well as personal, pressures to shape their reproductive decisions. The justification is usually based on public health needs. Debates surrounding modern public health crises, such as the spread of HIV infection, often use an adversarial model focused largely on balancing a presumed conflict between individual rights against community rights. This adversarial vision may well be due to the decline of widespread communicable disease, the rise of the medical profession, and the development of an individualistic, rights-based system of justice (Parmet, 1989). For many public health issues such as genetic testing and screening, however, individual interests may be in harmony with public interests, and thus cooperative models of governmental and individual action may be more appropriate (Bayer, 1989; Parmet, 1989; Gostin, Curran, & Clark, 1987; Shilts, 1987).

Historically, governments have viewed preventing disease and providing medical care as core functions, whether that entailed disease reporting and sanitary engineering or quarantine and health care (Parmet, 1985; Rosenkrantz, 1972). The police power of the state to take such measures seemed to be based on long-held doctrines that the use of property (and in turn, individual action) was limited by the extent to which it created a public nuisance (Schwartz, 1974). Even after the mid-nineteenth century, when federal constitutional law guarantees of individual rights were applied, public health regulation was viewed as largely immune from constitutional challenge (Tribe, 1988; Tushnet, 1988; Schwartz, 1974). Even draconian quarantine measures have been upheld on the basis that "*salus populi suprema lex*" (the safety of the people is the supreme law).[5] "The police power was, in short, the public's right to self-survival" (Parmet, 1989).

Where the public health hazards were "democratic," in other words, where they cut across class, race, ethnic, and gender

lines in the community, there was no apparent distinction between individual interests and community interests. When any
member of the community might be the next to fall ill, there
was a common need for defense against the spread of illness and
a common need for compassion for those afflicted. As disease
became viewed more as a sign of moral and spiritual failing,
however, those who imposed restrictions (who assumed themselves of superior character) began to feel safe from suffering
under such constraints themselves. This was particularly true as
immigration rose, and the foreign-language-speaking, often impoverished newcomers were viewed as a distinct group bringing
disease and moral impurity with them (Rosenkrantz, 1972; Rosenberg, 1962).

Courts eventually began to recognize that disease control
could be used abusively to oppress certain economic, racial, and
ethnic minorities, and slowly increased judicial scrutiny of
public health measures (Parmet, 1985). With their newfound
awareness, the courts needed a principle by which to distinguish
legitimate from illegitimate public health interests. The medi-
calization of health helped to provide that principle: Advances
in bacteriology and sanitation created a scientific basis for public
health policy, and this increased the delegation of public health
powers into the hands of scientifically trained individuals. Over
time this evolved into a policy requiring that individuals follow
the advice of medical professionals lest they be viewed as having
caused their own illness and threatened to make others ill as well
(Parmet, 1985; Rosenkrantz, 1972; Rosenberg, 1962).

As is discussed below, in the area of reproductive health the
courts have often adopted an adversarial model in which they
balance the right of the community to protect itself from individuals whose decisions threaten the health and makeup of
the next generation[6] (Bartrum, 1992; Johnsen, 1992; Oberman,
1992) against the individual's right to make reproductive decisions free of government coercion.[7] Limitation on the community's right (such as the "right" to require genetic screening) is
found only in those constitutional provisions designed to protect individuals against the excesses of government action: the
Fourth Amendment's protection against unreasonable searches;
the Fifth and Fourteenth Amendments' assurances of due pro-

cess and equal protection under the law; the First Amendment's protection of the exercise of religion; and the doctrine of fundamental rights with regard to marriage and procreation (Adelman, 1981). Yet ironically, it is in the area of reproduction where harmony may exist between public health and individual goals, obviating the need for such adversarial analysis (Johnsen, 1992).

As the story of Bree Walker Lampley demonstrates, there is strong public sentiment against bringing children into the world knowing they will suffer debilitating and painful illness. It is, however, the very people who make the choice whether to bring them into the world who will have the primary responsibility for their care and succor. Who better, then, to make the choice of whether to conceive such a child than the people who will be there to help the child, financially and emotionally, through every hospitalization or every physical therapy session.

As the Human Genome Project continues to identify the genetic risks we all face in procreation, genetic diagnosis and counseling will become an aspect of personal health for the entire community, not just certain members or certain ethnic groups. The development of tests for cystic fibrosis is particularly significant because it heralds an era in which the Caucasian population is potentially subject to genetic screening and governmental influence regarding reproductive choices. Until now, the population groups thus targeted have largely been racial and ethnic minorities who are still working toward full acceptance and effectiveness within the political community. The earlier vision of public health, in which the entire community viewed itself at general risk, could therefore replace the present vision, in which only certain groups are at risk. This in turn could restore the inherent safeguards necessary to make majoritarian politics a more reasonable way for the community to make choices concerning the implementation of widespread genetic screening programs, and reduce the temptation to view public health models of genetic screening as a battle between community interests and individual rights.

Unfortunately, this commonality of interests is rarely recognized in reproductive politics. Instead, manipulating women's reproductive choices to meet community perceptions of intergenerational need is a common phenomenon. While public interest in the size and composition of a population is certainly legitimate, it is not a sufficient justification for choosing the most interventionist and burdensome restrictions on women's freedom before seeking alternative solutions. The unusually interventionist population policies of China and Romania during the 1970s and 1980s illustrate the problem.

China's policy, still active in the 1990s, combines public information campaigns with tax and employment penalties for those urban women having more than one child and rural women having more than two. Those extreme costs are borne by women despite the fact that other means, such as enhanced education for girls, are powerful tools to meet public goals of reduced population growth without burdening women. Some argue that the urgency of the population growth in China required drastic measures with short-term returns. But the readiness with which the Chinese government chose to penalize women, rather than men, indicates a tendency to view women's bodies and reproductive propensities as legitimate tools of state policy.

The Romanian pro-natalist policies were equally interventionist. To ensure an adequate supply of labor for the postwar economy, women were forbidden access to contraceptives. Many were subjected to repeated pregnancy tests at their places of work. Those found pregnant were required to submit to follow-up examinations. A miscarriage would result in an investigation to determine if it had been induced. Induced miscarriage, of course, was a crime—not against the fetus, as is argued here in the United States, but against the state and the community. Once again, despite noninterventionist options for meeting state policy goals (such as increasing immigration from impoverished countries who have too many people to support), the community and government reaction was to look for a more immediate solution that entailed using women as a means to state ends.

Here in the United States, the Human Genome Project offers the prospect of an American-style debate over similar policies. Despite the rhetoric emphasizing the freedom to have children as a "fundamental" right (Robertson, 1986, 1983), the United

States has a long history of eugenic thinking and has often rushed to mold women's reproductive decisions to meet state policy goals. In the United States the first eugenic sterilization law was passed in Indiana in 1907; twenty-nine more would follow (Reilly, 1991). The 1924 Johnson Act premised immigration policy on racist theories about the relative merits of peoples originating from various parts of Europe. Even Margaret Sanger, most influential of the early supporters of access to birth control, endorsed government offering monetary rewards to those who would be "unfit" parents if they would agree to sterilization (Gordon, 1990). More recently, state legislatures have begun to seriously debate whether to offer financial incentives—ranging from threatened withdrawal of existing social benefits to actual cash grants—to poor or drug-addicted women who choose to have a long-term contraceptive placed in their bodies. Several courts have ordered women convicted of child abuse to choose between a jail sentence and the implantation of the same, long-acting contraceptive (NYT, 1993; Southwick, 1992; UPI, 1993, 1992). Consistent with these interventionist approaches to furthering eugenic policies, American prosecutors and courts have shown a tendency to attempt to further the more general state goal of child protection by way of forced caesarean sections and prosecution of pregnant addicts.[8]

With the prospect of better predictive diagnosis of disorder, there will be the temptation to ask whether we as a nation have an obligation to future generations to minimize their burdens, both personal and economic, from the presence of physical or mental disorders among them. Further, if the decision is made that such an obligation exists, there will be the temptation to protect those generations through state interventionist policies. Though the politics of abortion and the right-to-life movement probably forestall drastic policies such as that adopted in China, numerous indirect pressures could be brought to bear. These range from public service messages, to mandatory genetic testing as a condition for the granting of a marriage license, to differential insurance coverage in the semiprivate and public insurance markets.

It might be argued that we owe nothing to future generations; after all, they consist of people who do not yet exist, may never exist, and cannot be known to us now as individuals. Furthermore, any rights they might have to protection are nonreciprocal (because they can do nothing for those of us currently living) and unenforceable. Indeed, our very actions taken on their behalf would change the genetic makeup of that future generation, thus resulting in the paradox of our taking actions on behalf of individuals who might well cease to exist as a result of those actions (Parfit, 1984, 1981).

This is an overly simplistic view, though, at least as it is premised on an atomistic, individualistic view of rights and obligations. Those future people, as yet undefined and unknowable, may be viewed as part of our moral community because they will eventually become sentient, actual people, linked to us in time if not necessarily in space. Looked at collectively, "[society] is a partnership in all science . . . art . . . virtue, and . . . perfection. As the ends of such a partnership cannot be obtained in many generations, it becomes a partnership not only between those who are living, but between those who are living, those who are dead, and those who are to be born" (Burke, 1959). As members of a common moral community, we who are living ought to abide by that implicit social contract because our obligation to the future stems from our debt to the past. One commentator likens this notion to the Japanese concept of *"on"* (roughly, obligation), in which "[o]ne makes payment on '*on*' to one's parents by giving equally good or better rearing to one's children. The obligations one has to one's children are merely subsumed under '*on*' to one's parents" (Benedict, 1946).

Accepting the notion of obligation to future generations does not, however, imply limitless duties. It would appear excessive to argue that we who are living owe them more than we owe ourselves. The reason for their claim on us (that they will be living) is no more pressing than the claim we make upon ourselves. After all, we too are living. Furthermore, their claims upon us are still conditioned upon their coming into existence and choosing to press a claim. Our claims upon ourselves are not conditional; they are already real. Thus, to some extent, the claims of members of the current generation upon the resources and liberties of society are superior to those of future generations.

Given this limitation, one might realistically claim that the current generation, as a community, owes future generations a degree of restraint, such as a willingness to refrain from doing things we know will be significantly harmful. But even this does not go far enough. After all, we do some significantly harmful things to ourselves because there are economic or moral imperatives that drive our decisions. Each new interstate highway harms the aesthetic and biological values of the terrain in the name of economic development. To borrow again from the jargon of tort law, then, we can probably argue that the current generation owes a duty to refrain from negligent acts harming future generations. Such negligence can roughly be defined as engaging in behaviors that put future generations at an unreasonable risk of harm in the light of the purported benefits to be accrued by so acting. And, again as in tort law, we can look to custom as a rough and ready, though by no means irrebuttable, presumption of reasonableness. To the extent that we treat future generations no differently than we treat ourselves, we have probably fulfilled our obligations. Our own sense of the fairness of the trade-offs we are making for ourselves provides the best available guide to how future generations are likely to view similar choices. Boiled down to a formula, we who are now living probably owe those who will be living a world perhaps different in kind but not significantly worse in degree than the one we ourselves occupy. Thus, until we demand for ourselves a world free of all avoidable genetic, or indeed physical, disorders, we can hardly be said to owe the same to future generations.

The question then must be asked, how can or should we create a world for ourselves and for future generations that minimizes our burdens? The answer must be that we make sacrifices and trade-offs. The public health doctrine of quarantine requires a sacrifice on the part of the infectious person for the benefit of the community as a whole. It involves a trade-off between individual autonomy and community well-being. But the fact that such a trade-off can be made does not suggest that it need not meet minimal standards of justice. Vaccination refusals are permitted in order to honor our commitment to principles of bodily integrity, parental authority, and free exercise of religion. Tuberculosis isolation is chosen only after proven medicines and directly observed therapy fail to halt the spread of infection. And quarantine is completely eschewed when, as with the epidemic of HIV infection, it would entail an enormous, lifelong burden on those who are infected and only marginally improve upon other methods of protecting the public interest in controlling the spread of the disease.

Similarly, with regard to eugenic uses of information emerging from the Human Genome Project, any sacrifice demanded of specific individuals for the benefit of current and future generations must meet standards of justice. It is pointless to try to ensure *inter*generational justice by violating principles of *intra*generational justice. Looked at over a continuum of time, such a trade-off does nothing to further the goal of achieving a morally responsible community across generations. And that in turn means a just distribution of sacrifice not only between generations but within generations.

One influential concept of justice discussed among law professors today is that presented in John Rawls's *A Theory of Justice*. Rawls sets out a social contract procedure designed to arrive at those principles of justice that appear imperative. He argues that valid principles of justice are those we would agree upon if each of us were to freely and impartially consider the situation from a standpoint removed from any actual society (the "original position") and from which we each bargain with others similarly rendered impartial by virtue of this "veil of ignorance." Ignorant of our own biological attributes or position in whatever sort of society we were to create, Rawls argues that rational bargainers would inevitably agree upon a certain set of principles (Rawls, 1971). Concerned with utilitarianism's propensity for looking at maximization of total social good with little attention to its distribution, Rawls concludes that there is an inevitable set of principles of justice that any set of rational negotiators would agree upon. They would, he argues, create a society based upon permitting the maximum amount of liberty for each individual compatible with liberty for all, and in which inequalities in primary social goods (income, rights, opportunities) are allowed only if they ultimately inure to the benefit of everyone. This latter principle he refines to mean that inequalities are tolerable only if they most enhance the position of the least advantaged.

How can this concept guide decisions about fulfilling our collective duty to future generations, particularly with regard to women's obligations to fashion their reproductive lives to meet current community goals about the size and structure of future populations? Although Rawlsian principles of justice cannot be blindly applied to measure the merit of a particular social program within an actual society that was not derived through his thought experiment, it can provide some clue as to whether, in an ideal world, such a program would be tolerated.

Few could argue with the proposition that women are consistently disadvantaged in society. State policies that rely on control of women's bodies and reproductive decision-making to promote community preferences for future generations free of genetic disorder would certainly not appear to maximize each person's liberty consistent with the liberty of others. Rather, they single out one group, fertile women, for special restriction of liberty on behalf of community interests. Further, this curtailment of liberty does not inure to the benefit of the least advantaged; rather, it inures to the benefit of the community as a whole (assuming that having fewer persons with genetic disorders in the population really is a benefit) at the expense of the least advantaged.

The result, then, is that fertile women are conscripted to serve the reproductive preferences of the leadership in the community. In *Planned Parenthood of Pennsylvania v. Casey*,[9] Justice Blackmun argues in his dissent that this is an equal protection violation, created by abortion restrictions:

> By restricting the right to terminate pregnancies, the State conscripts women's bodies into its service, forcing women to continue their pregnancies, suffer the pains of childbirth, and in most instances, provide years of maternal care. The State does not compensate women for their services; instead, it assumes that they owe this duty as a matter of course. This assumption—that women can simply be forced to accept the "natural" status and incidents of

motherhood—appears to rest upon a conception of women's role that has triggered the protection of the Equal Protection Clause.

The inequalities in reproductive choice should be no more tolerable when proposed as simply making women accountable to the public for their reproductive decisions. Such accountability can range from the seemingly benign mandatory testing for genetic conditions (in order to ready a woman to make a decision about reproduction) to the draconian forced sterilization of the genetically "unfit," such as was authorized in well over half of the United States during this very century.

Rawlsian analyses of justice aside, there are good and traditional legal grounds upon which to criticize proposals that make women accountable to the public for their reproductive decisions. Faced with a credible public policy, enforcement mechanisms must nonetheless be tested against distinct criteria. First, does the enforcement infringe upon a fundamental right or a protected class of persons? If so, does the public policy represent a compelling governmental purpose? Is the chosen enforcement mechanism the most effective, least restrictive alternative? It is worth noting that this legal formulation resembles elements of the Rawlsian principles of justice. It tolerates infringements upon individual liberty only when for a compelling purpose (here somewhat broader than the Rawlsian concept that only maintenance of liberty for others qualifies as such as purpose). Further, it incorporates a protection against inequalities in rights or benefits when they disproportionately burden a disadvantaged class (somewhat more tolerant of inequality than Rawls, who permits it only when it benefits the disadvantaged class).

Manipulation of reproductive decisions does infringe upon a fundamental right. The right to procreate is grounded in both personal liberty and the integrity of the family unit and is viewed as fundamental to notions of ordered liberty and justice (Robertson, 1992, 1990, 1986, 1983). Although the *Casey* decision abandons the language of "fundamental" rights with regard to abortion decisions, it does leave untouched—for the moment—the line of cases implying that the decision to *have* a child is fundamentally protected under the due process and liberty clauses.[10] And the grounding of this right in the early-twentieth-century decisions concerning family autonomy (such as parental control over childhood education) argues in favor of interpreting the right to procreate as not only the right to *have* children but also the right to make some choices about what *kind* of children one will have (Robertson, 1986, 1983).

Given, then, that reproduction holds an exalted place among implicit constitutional rights, can state interests in reducing the number of children born with genetic disorders pass muster? Most means to promote this goal will impair women's reproductive freedom. Even mandatory screening laws impose a burden. They require individuals to learn things about themselves they may have no wish to know and potentially threaten their economic security by putting them at risk of social stigmatization as well as employment and insurance discrimination. These laws can, in the end, have a chilling effect on the exercise of the right to procreate. Past experience coupled with pilot projects on cystic fibrosis carrier screening in the United Kingdom and the United States demonstrate that such screening efforts will be directed primarily at women rather than at men or at couples (U.S. Congress, 1992). Thus, even mandatory screening programs place a burden on the exercise of a fundamental right by women, a group that is historically disadvantaged.[11] If states wish to reduce the purported burden of genetic disorders, the goal must be compelling and the means chosen must be the most effective and the least restrictive possible. The implementation of mandatory screening fails to meet these criteria.

The goal of reducing genetic disorder in the population may be founded upon several propositions. First, it may reflect an economic concern that genetic disorder is costly. Second, it may reflect a desire to reduce human suffering. Third, it may be part of a teleological scheme for moving the population toward some "better" level of species functioning. None of these goals, however, is effectively served by screening laws, let alone by more drastic or harsh measures. While genetic disorders impose costs on the population through cost-sharing health and social welfare programs, they do not approach the costs incurred for other disorders, including those caused by trauma (crime, accident, workplace injury), undetected or untreated disease, and even illiteracy. Human suffering is far greater due to malnutrition, lack of shelter, and community violence than to relatively rare genetic disorders. And improvement of the population's capacity to engage in intellectually demanding work would take place far more quickly via universal literacy than via the reduction in the number of individuals with Down syndrome. State interests in "improving" the population and reducing suffering can be met far more effectively in areas having little or nothing to do with reproductive decision-making.

Voluntary screening programs, whether directed at women exclusively or not, offer a means of enhancing personal liberty (by making it easier to make an informed choice about procreation) while simultaneously serving governmental objectives that would otherwise go unmet. Mandatory education about basic genetics and the availability of screening services, like hygiene courses in high school, can empower women without manipulating them. Focusing on the personal liberty of those making reproductive decisions, rather than on the dubious public goal of eugenic cleansing of the gene pool, puts limits on the techniques that can be used by the government to promote genetic screening or to penalize women who make unpopular decisions regarding procreation in the face of genetic risk. It puts women's bodies back in the service of their own life goals, rather than the service of the government's most immediate objectives.

Conclusion

The Human Genome Project promises to vastly increase the amount of knowledge available to us concerning the likely birth outcomes of our children. History demonstrates that the state will be sorely tempted to use that knowledge for eugenic purposes, employing the most interventionist methods possible, if only because historically there has been little regard for women making reproductive decisions on their own behalf and for their own interests. Rather, women's reproductive decisions have consistently been viewed as being made for the benefit of others, whether their husbands, their families, or the state. Yet since women will inevitably be the main targets of genetic information, screening, and planning, as well as the primary caretakers of those born with genetic disorders, justice dictates that increased freedom of action accompany this increased degree of responsibility. That freedom includes adequate information about the availability of genetic testing, sensitive counseling and guidance in its use, and equal support for pregnancy termination or continuation.

It is essential that we take advantage of the current state of constitutional law that has allowed pro-natalist aspects of reproductive freedom to rise to the level of a fundamental right. With this official nod from the Supreme Court, it is possible to resist most state interventions on the basis that they unduly burden unfettered exercise of this right. Overall, it is worth remembering that we do not owe our children or our children's children an endless sacrifice of personal interests. Intergenerational justice dictates that we leave future generations no worse off than we are ourselves. While we might aspire to more, we cannot demand it.

In the end, the legal response to expanded reproductive genetic testing will determine who controls the technology. The assumptions we make, for example, about causing or preventing harm may well affect the development of relevant law. To the extent that women's choices, autonomous or otherwise, are viewed as "causing" harm, those choices will be subject to significant limitation. If the passage of a deleterious gene from a parent to a child is considered "causing" harm, then women's decisions about genetic screening and pregnancy termination could well be the subject of state interest. On the other hand, if these are viewed as decisions simply not to "prevent" harm, the decisions are more likely to be left unfettered. Of course, the biggest risk in the light of expanded opportunities for genetic testing is the development of an affirmative duty to prevent all avoidable harms to future children from whatever cause. This is exactly the sort of theory used in numerous forced caesarean and fetal protection policy cases.

Both providers and consumers must recognize there are limits on control over reproduction and the duty to rescue members of the next generation from the results of the genetic lottery. The expansion of genetic testing may give the impression we can and should take complete control and responsibility for the results of birth. But in the end we must recognize that conditions beyond our knowledge or grasp may cause results that we cannot control. Law cannot change this biological reality.

NOTES

1. 492 U.S. 490 (1989).
2. 112 S. Ct. 2791 (1992).
3. 500 U.S. 173 (1991).
4. For a detailed discussion of wrongful birth and wrongful life suits, see Ellen Wright Clayton, "What the Law Says about Reproductive Genetic Testing and What It Doesn't," chapter 8 in this book.
5. *Seavey v. Preble*, 64 Me. 120 (1874).
6. *Buck v. Bell*, 274 U.S. 200 (1927).
7. *Skinner v. Oklahoma*, 316 U.S. 535 (1942); *Griswold v. Connecticut*, 381 U.S. 479 (1965); *Eisenstadt v. Baird*, 405 U.S. 438 (1972); *Roe v. Wade*, 410 U.S. 113 (1973).
8. See, e.g., *State v. Gray*, No. 90–1986 (Ohio Feb. 12, 1992); *Johnson v. State*, No. 77, 831 (Fla. Jul. 23, 1992); *Reyes v. Superior Court*, 75 Cal. App. 3rd 214 (1977); *People v. Hardy*, No. 128458 (Mich. Ct. App., April 1, 1991); *State v. Gethers*, 585 So.2d 1140 (Fla. Fourth D.C.A. 1991); *Welch v. Commonwealth*, No. 90-CA-1189-MR (Ky. Ct. App., Feb. 7, 1992); *State v. Carter*, No. 90–2261 (Fla. First D.C.A., August 13, 1992); *People v. Morabito*, (N.Y. Cnty. Ct. Ontario Sept. 24, 1992); *In re A.C.*, 573 A.2d 1235 (D.C., 1990).
9. 112 S. Ct. 2791, 2846–47 (1992).
10. Of course, the Supreme Court has not explicitly considered whether there is a positive right to procreate. It has, however, considered a wide range of related issues, including the right of the state to interfere with procreative ability by forcible sterilization (*Skinner v. Oklahoma*, 316 U.S. 535 (1942)), the right of individuals to prevent conception or continued pregnancy (*Eisenstadt v. Baird*, 405 U.S. 438 (1972); *Griswold v. Connecticut*, 381 U.S. 479 (1965); *Roe v. Wade*, 410 U.S. 113 (1973); *Planned Parenthood of Pennsylvania v. Casey*, 112 S. Ct. 2791 (1992)); and the right of individuals to rear children and to form nontraditional families (*Loving v. Virginia*, 388 U.S. 1 (1967); *Meyer v. Nebraska*, 292 U.S. 390 (1923); *Pierce v. Society of Sisters*, 288 U.S. 510 (1925)).
11. *Craig v. Boren*, 429 U.S. 190 (1976); *Frontiero v. Richardson*, 411 U.S. 677 (1973).

BIBLIOGRAPHY

ADELMAN, C. S. (1981). The constitutionality of mandatory genetic screening statutes. *Case Western Reserve Law Review, 31*, 897–948.

AMERICAN Political Network. (1993, January 25). Clinton lifts five restrictions. *The Abortion Report.*

BARTRUM, T. E. (1992). Birth control as a condition of probation—A new weapon in the war against child abuse. *Kentucky Law Journal, 80,* 1037–1053.

BAYER, R. (1989). *Private acts, social consequences: AIDS and the politics of public health.* New York: The Free Press.

BENEDICT, R. (1946). *The chrysanthemum and the sword.* Boston: Houghton Mifflin.

BENN, P. A., Hsu, L. Y. F., Carlson, A., et al. (1985). The centralized prenatal genetics screening program of New York City: III, the first 7,000 cases. *American Journal of Medical Genetics, 20,* 369–384.

BURKE, E. (1959). *Reflections of the French Revolution.* New York: Holt Rinehart Winston.

CLAYTON, E. W. (1993). What the law says about reproductive genetic testing and what it doesn't. In K. H. Rothenberg & E. J. Thomson (Eds.), *Women and Prenatal Testing: Facing the Challenges of Genetic Technology.* Columbus, OH: Ohio State University Press.

FADEN, R. R., Chwalow, A. J., Quaid, K., et al. (1987). Prenatal screening and pregnant women's attitudes toward the abortion of defective fetuses. *American Journal of Public Health, 77,* 288–290.

GOLBUS, M. S., Loughman, W. D., Epstein, C. J., et al. (1979). Prenatal diagnosis in 3000 amniocenteses. *New England Journal of Medicine, 300,* 157–163.

GORDON, L. (1990). *Woman's body, woman's right: Birth control in America.* New York: Penguin Books.

GOSTIN, L. O., Curran, W. J., & Clark, M. (1987). The case against compulsory casefinding in controlling AIDS—Testing, screening and reporting. *American Journal of Law and Medicine, 12*(1), 7–53.

JOHNSEN, D. (1992). Shared interests: Promoting healthy births without sacrificing women's liberty. *Hastings Law Journal, 43,* 569–614.

NATIONAL Abortion Rights Action League. (1992). *Who decides?* Washington, DC: NARAL.

NEW York Times Editorial Desk. (1993, February 12). Sterilization and unfit mothers. *New York Times.*

OBERMANN, M. (1992). Sex, drugs, pregnancy, and the law: Rethinking the problems of pregnant women who use drugs. *Hastings Law Journal, 43,* 505.

PARFIT, D. (1981). *Energy policy and the further future.* College Park, MD: Center for Philosophy and Public Policy.

PARFIT, D. (1984). *Reasons and persons.* Oxford: Clarendon Press.

PARMET, W. E. (1985). AIDS and quarantine: The revival of an archaic doctrine. *Hofstra Law Review, 14*(1), 137–162.

PARMET, W. E. (1989). Legal rights and communicable disease: AIDS, the police power, and individual liberty. *Journal of Health Politics, Policy and Law, 14*(4), 741–771.

RAWLS, J. (1971). *A theory of justice.* Cambridge, MA: Belknap Press.

REILLY, P. (1991). *The surgical solution.* Baltimore: Johns Hopkins University Press.

ROBERTSON, J. A. (1983). Procreative liberty and the control of conception, pregnancy, and childbirth. *Virginia Law Review, 69*, 405–464.

ROBERTSON, J. A. (1986). Embryos, families, and procreative liberty: The legal structure of the new reproduction. *Southern California Law Review, 59*, 942-1041.

ROBERTSON, J. A. (1990). Procreative liberty and human genetics. *Emory Law Journal, 39*, 697–719.

ROBERTSON, J. A. (1992). Legal issues in genetic testing. In *The genome, ethics, and the law: Issues in genetic testing.* Washington, DC: American Association for the Advancement of Science.

ROSENBERG, C. (1962). *The cholera years: The United States in 1832, 1849, and 1866.* Chicago, IL: University of Chicago Press.

ROSENKRANTZ, B. (1972). *Public health and the state: Changing views in Massachusetts, 1842–1936.* Cambridge, MA: Harvard University Press.

SCHWARTZ, B. (1974). *The law in America.* New York: McGraw-Hill.

SHILTS, R. (1987). *And the band played on: Politics, people and the AIDS epidemic.* New York: St. Martin's.

SINGER, E. (1991). Public attitudes toward genetic testing. *Population Research and Policy Review, 10*, 235–255.

SOUTHWICK, K. (1992, August 2). Use Norplant, don't go to jail. *San Francisco Chronicle.*

TRIBE, L. (1988). *American constitutional law* (2nd ed.). Mineola, NY: Foundation Press.

TUSHNET, M. (1988). *Red, white and blue: A critical analysis of constitutional law.* Cambridge, MA: Harvard University Press.

UNITED Press International. (1992, November 14). Judge finds no legal precedent for ordering contraception.

UNITED Press International. (1993, February 11). ACLU will challenge Norplant sentence.

u.s. Congress, Office of Technology Assessment (Biological Applications Program). (1992). Cystic fibrosis: Implications for carrier screening. Washington, DC: United States Government Publishing Office

Wertz, D. C., Rosenfield, J. M., Janes, S. R., et al. (1991). Attitudes toward abortion among parents of children with cystic fibrosis. *American Journal of Public Health, 81*(8), 922–996.

8

What the Law Says about Reproductive Genetic Testing and What It Doesn't

ELLEN WRIGHT CLAYTON

Health care providers are usually asked to detect diseases in order to protect previously healthy individuals from becoming ill and to cure those who have become ill. Diagnosis, in these cases, is pursued in order to permit therapeutic intervention directed at returning people to health. This model, however, cannot be usefully applied to reproductive genetic testing. Because genetic disorders are inherited, fetuses or children who are found to be affected have never been "normal." They may be asymptomatic, but they are not the same as other individuals who have a different genetic makeup. There are also limits on what can be done once genetic disease is detected. Not only is it impossible to change one's genes, but there often are no truly curative or even largely ameliorative interventions for those disorders. In particular, there are very few effective therapies that must, or can, be begun in the prenatal or neonatal period.

As a result, while some people want reproductive genetic tests so that they can prepare themselves for the medical problems their children may have, the overriding reason these tests are offered and used is to prevent the birth of children with genetic disorders. The desire to use reproductive genetic testing for "prevention" will probably continue to play a major role, even when effective therapy becomes readily available, because

131

of the financial, emotional, and practical burdens associated with medical treatment.

The options available to avoid the birth of a child with genetic disorders depends on the point at which the woman and her partner are in the procreative process. If the woman is not yet pregnant, she and her partner may be able to use sperm or egg donation or may simply choose to avoid having children altogether. Once she is pregnant, however, the only way to avoid having children affected with these disorders is to use abortion—either selectively, if the disorder can be diagnosed prenatally, or generally.

Public discourse about reproductive genetic testing is heavily influenced and ultimately divided by the connections made between this sort of testing and the already controversial procedures affecting procreation such as artificial insemination by donor and egg donation on the one hand, and contraception and abortion on the other. People from many different political and religious perspectives are concerned about the use of reproductive genetic testing. Some, who profess to believe in a "right to life," argue that these tests are objectionable because all life is sacred, and they fear that the tests interfere with and may potentially threaten the lives of fetuses. Others view as immoral any form of (or influence upon) procreation besides unprotected coitus, a stance that excludes any use of genetic tests or new reproductive technologies (Congregation, 1990).

By contrast, some feminists and advocates for the rights of the disabled—including some of the contributors to this book—worry that the use of reproductive genetic tests may decrease our society's already poor tolerance of difference and may shift the onus of having a child with a genetic disorder even further away from society, onto families and in particular women instead (Rothman, 1986; Lippman, 1991). Other commentators point out that social structures that make it difficult to care for sick children can also make it difficult for potential parents to decline testing. There is little evidence, however, that legislators respond to the voices of these latter groups of critics.

At the other extreme, some people adhere to eugenic notions that the birth of children with genetic disorders places an inappropriate burden on society. The long history of such beliefs in this country is evidenced by the thousands of people who have been involuntarily sterilized in the United States in this century.[1] While present day eugenicists may not be willing to advocate openly for mandatory testing, contraception, and abortion because these notions are too unseemly in the wake of the well-known abuses here and abroad earlier in this century, they may support making testing widely available for the "public good" (Cunningham, 1990). And at some level, one has to acknowledge that reproductive genetic testing would not be made available, especially at public expense, unless people actually relied on the results to avoid having children affected by genetic disorders. The reassurance that most people feel when they get "good news" would certainly not be enough by itself to support the widespread application of these tests.

Still another group asserts that individual families ought to be able to make informed reproductive choices to suit their own goals. This sort of argument fits comfortably within the deference paid, if primarily only in words, to notions of autonomy and family privacy. Rhetoric of this kind is important, however, because of its prominent place in our public discourse.

These varying views have quite different implications in terms of policy that have the potential for conflicting with each other in fundamental ways. Thus, it is somewhat surprising that a large body of statutory, regulatory, and case law exists dealing directly and indirectly with the provision of genetic services. Many of these laws have evolved through state legislation, although the federal government has also played an important role. A close look reveals that there is indeed wide variation among the states in their approaches to reproductive genetic testing, with many states also having internal inconsistencies in their policies regarding genetics. In addition, the federal government has changed its position rather dramatically in the past 15 years. Taken together, these differences and conflicts demonstrate that there is little agreement about the appropriate use of prenatal genetic technologies.

The discussion that follows begins with an analysis of the present state of the law, looking first at cases, statutes, and regulations that directly address the provision of genetic services. Many of those statutes and regulations deal with issues of access, most commonly by setting up state programs to provide some sort of genetic information and services to their citizens, and less frequently by requiring insurers to pay for the services. In addition, there is a burgeoning body of case law in which children with genetic disorders and their parents sue their health care providers arguing that the providers failed to supply adequate information for the parents regarding genetic risk. The families have often been at least partially successful in pursuing these claims, giving physicians added incentive to perform genetic testing and provide counseling. Some state legislatures have undermined these privately generated pressures by passing statutes that limit or eliminate families' causes of action.

The other major body of law directly affecting reproductive genetic testing is that dealing with abortion, since the main reason people use prenatal diagnosis at present is to allow them to choose whether to terminate the pregnancy if they receive an undesired result. Most current abortion statutes say little about this justification for wanting to terminate pregnancy. Their relative silence may have a substantial impact on reproductive genetic testing in the future, given the erosion of the United States Constitution's protection of the right to choose abortion. If states are once again allowed to regulate the reasons for which women may terminate pregnancies, it will be important to draw a distinction between those modes of testing that influence the decision of whether to conceive at all, and prenatal diagnosis, which almost inherently entails the possibility of abortion.

Access to Genetic Services

Although health care traditionally has been thought to be the responsibility of the states, the federal government has taken an increasingly prominent role in this area, largely by using money as an incentive to the states to provide health care services. Congress in the 1970s responded to the development of the "new genetics" by passing a variety of laws, culminating in the National Genetic Diseases Act in 1976, which provided separate funding for grants to the states to establish programs providing genetic services.[2]

In the 1980s, this practice changed. To begin with, the separate funding provided under the National Genetic Diseases Act was repealed. Those programs were instead included within a special set-aside within the Maternal and Child Health Services Block Grant. The present statute has two important limitations. The Secretary of Health and Human Services can award support only to "special projects of regional and national significance, research, and training." More important, it provides that programs directed at genetic disease must compete for funding with initiatives for maternal and child health, children with special needs, individuals with hemophilia, and newborn screening,[3] all at a time of decreased federal support for domestic programs. In addition, the detailed regulations promulgated under the National Genetic Diseases Act, which had made clear that a broad range of services were to be made available and which made no reference to abortion,[4] were repealed in 1988.[5]

The regulations that now govern speak of genetic testing only in the most general terms and make clear that those funds cannot be used to pay for abortion unless the pregnancy either presents a threat to the life of the woman or was the result of rape or incest,[6] neither of which is likely to be the case for abortions for genetic indications. Under these restrictions, women who are poor or who have no way to pay for abortion can, theoretically, have prenatal diagnosis paid for with federal funds. But unless they are able to come up with some other funds to pay for abortion, they can use these technologies only to obtain reassurance or to prepare for what is to come.

What remains of the grant-making authority conferred by the National Genetic Diseases Act is that the Secretary of Health and Human Services is empowered to fund research, to educate professionals and the public, and to develop programs "for the diagnosis, control, and treatment of genetic diseases." The source of such funds is not clear, however, and preference is to be given in any event to sickle-cell anemia and thalassemia.[7]

The federal government does provide some genetic services itself. The Public Health Service, for example, is directed to "provide voluntary testing, diagnosis, counseling, and treatment of individuals respecting genetic diseases."[8] Moreover, some members of the armed services and their families can obtain genetic services as well.[9] CHAMPUS, the health insurance for military personnel and their families, for example, pays for prenatal diagnosis of both genetic and developmental disorders if the women is 35 years old or older or had rubella during the first trimester of pregnancy, or if the couple has a previous child with or a family history of a congenital abnormality. Its coverage explicitly excludes "routine or demand" prenatal diagnosis or tests to determine the sex or paternity of the child.[10] Moreover, at least as of July, 1990, CHAMPUS covered the expense of most abortions,[11] so that prenatal diagnosis would be a practical option for those personnel. Many veterans and their families, however, cannot obtain abortions at government expense in this setting.[12] Thus, there is some, but incomplete, support at the federal level for enabling individuals to use the new genetic technologies.

The states, which have the primary responsibility for matters of health, vary greatly in their approaches to genetic services. (The details of those approaches are summarized in table 1 found in the appendix to this chapter.) Several state legislatures passed statutes providing for statewide genetics programs. Many of these were enacted in the heyday of the mid- to late 1970s, although California has revisited the topic several times, including passing several laws in the past two years. Some of the statutes are quite elaborate, providing in great detail, for example, that the services are voluntary and that the results are confidential.[13] Others are quite brief, saying nothing at all about protection of the interests of the potential counselees.[14] Indeed, some legislatures seem almost to have added statewide genetic services as an afterthought to their newborn screening laws,[15] statutes that themselves have often been the object of little legislative attention (Clayton, 1992). Other states have created genetics programs by regulation, without a specific enabling statute.[16]

Of particular interest is the fact that several states have established programs to provide prenatal diagnosis, most often by statute,[17] but occasionally by regulation.[18] Some of those states, however, have imposed substantial restrictions on the use of prenatal diagnosis. Minnesota and Missouri, for example, will provide testing in many instances but abortion rarely if at all.[19] Tennessee, which otherwise has a quite expansive program, provides that prenatal diagnosis will not be funded unless it would lead to treatment for either the pregnant woman or the child, stating that "the use of this program to abort unborn children is against the public policy of the state of Tennessee."[20]

A number of states have taken a more piecemeal approach to the provision of genetic services. To give a few examples, Pennsylvania provides funds to Jefferson Medical College to develop a program for Tay-Sachs disease, including counseling and "genetic diagnostic services."[21] Other states have directed that genetic screening be provided for families of individuals with mental disabilities.[22] Still another approach is to require that applicants for marriage licenses be given information about genetic disorders and where to be tested.[23] Finally, Kansas still requires that parents be given information about sickle-cell screening when their children enter school, despite the fact that children of that age are not the appropriate targets of genetic screening.[24]

States ensure access to genetic services not only by acting as direct providers or by paying for the services outright in programs that are specifically directed at genetics, but also by requiring others to pay for testing when it is provided by health care professionals in the private sector. Washington, Minnesota, and California require at least some insurers who provide maternity benefits to include prenatal diagnostic tests within the benefits package.[25] Louisiana mandates that those insurers who cover the care of people with cleft lip and palate include genetic assessment and counseling within the benefits provided, a service that that state's insurers apparently are not required to offer to individuals with any other heritable disorder.[26]

Finally, several states cover prenatal diagnosis under their program of medical assistance either directly as a matter of statute or by including such testing within their definition of family planning services.[27] The latter course has been risky for state family planning programs, which typically rely heavily on federal money. Adopting such an expansive definition of family planning appeared to conflict directly with the Bush administration's bans against mentioning abortion or providing anything more than emergency prenatal care once pregnancy has been diagnosed,[28] restrictions that the Supreme Court upheld in *Rust v. Sullivan*,[29] but that were rescinded by President Clinton's executive order in January, 1993.

Analysis of the statutes and regulations that address genetic services suggests that there is little consensus about these programs. Many state legislatures and administrative agencies have attempted to extend reproductive genetic testing and counseling to their citizens through both direct provision of services and financial subsidy. Often these governmental institutions have devoted limited attention to the implications of such services, however. Relatively few statutes, for example, contain provisions for such fundamental protections as confidentiality and voluntary participation.

In addition, not all states appear to think that such services are desirable. Some states like Tennessee limit the services that they will provide. State legislatures have expressed ambivalence toward, if not disapproval of, genetic testing in other ways as well, some of which are discussed in the next section. And a number of states have been entirely silent on the subject, suggesting that these states provide genetic testing and counseling to their citizens, if at all, by relying upon their broad mandates to provide for the health of their population. It seems likely that many of these states simply do not supply those services.

Wrongful Birth and Wrongful Life

Federal and state statutes and rules focusing on genetic services are not the only bodies of law that affect the provision of genetic testing and counseling. Such activities come well within our society's current notions of health care and so are subject to the laws of medical malpractice. In the past 25 years, children with genetic disorders and their families have filed a large number of lawsuits in which they allege that their health care providers inappropriately failed to supply sufficient genetic information. Most commentators and courts now agree that such cases can be divided into two broad categories. The first are the claims of the parents, which are designated as causes of action for "wrongful birth." The second are the claims of the affected children themselves, which are now termed "wrongful life" suits (Andrews, 1987; Wright, 1978).

Both sets of claims have essentially the same elements. The first is that the parents did not receive the relevant genetic information because of a health care provider's negligence. Negligence has a special definition in the legal system. It means not sloppiness or carelessness, but failure to meet the governing standard of care. This standard differs somewhat from state to state, but determining it usually involves asking whether the physician who was sued did something that other reasonable practitioners would not have done. Although the "reasonable practitioner" standard sounds straightforward, it can be elusive in practice. It almost invariably requires that the injured person obtain expert testimony verifying that the physician's care was inappropriate. The plaintiff's ability to provide this proof can be impeded by limitations on who can testify. In particular, the expert often must practice the same specialty as, and in a similar location to, the doctor being sued.[30] Where this is true, an injured party may have difficulty finding a physician who is willing to testify against another practitioner whom she may know or from whom she may get referrals.

There are numerous ways in which a physician's negligence can prevent parents from getting appropriate information. Most commonly, the problem occurs in diagnosis. The physician can fail to realize that the couple is at increased risk, either by neglecting to take a genetic or even ethnic history,[31] by not recognizing the implications of the history they did take,[32] or by failing to make a diagnosis of heritable disease in a child previously born to the couple.[33] Sometimes problems occur in the testing process—samples are mishandled or lost, for example[34]—so that a diagnosis is not made. Less frequently, physicians appropriately determine the genetic risk but fail to inform the family adequately of the consequences. Such claims ought to be treated as suits asserting lack of informed consent to childbearing,[35] although one court specifically rejected such an approach, stating that there had been no "affirmative violation of the plaintiff mother's physical integrity."[36]

If the family can show that their provider deviated from the standard of care, they must then show that the negligence caused them to suffer legally cognizable injury. For causation they must allege that had they been given the appropriate information, they would have chosen not to have the child. Where genetic disease was not discovered in an earlier child or where there was a problem in carrier screening, the couple need say only that had they been properly informed, they would have no more children at all or that they would have achieved conception in some other manner, such as using artificial insemination by donor, if that would have avoided the risk. Where the negligence allegedly occurred after the woman was already pregnant, she must say that she would have aborted the pregnancy either with or without prenatal diagnosis.

In some cases, alleging that the negligent failure to inform during pregnancy occurred prior to the Supreme Court's decision in *Roe v. Wade*,[37] the courts refused to permit recovery—in part on the ground that the woman could not have obtained a legal abortion even had she known.[38] This may become an issue again should some of the states succeed in their efforts to impose severe restrictions on access to abortion. Were that to occur, courts who favored families' claims in these circumstances might well return to a strategy used by some judges in the past who pointed out that prior to 1973 a woman who lived in a restrictive state could travel to states in which abortions were legally available.[39]

While the existence of negligence and causation are essential elements of a suit alleging inadequate disclosure of genetic risk, such issues have not given rise to much reported appellate litigation, perhaps because they fit fairly comfortably within a traditional medical malpractice analysis. The major source of contention has been whether the birth of a child with a genetic disorder gives rise to any sort of legally compensable injury. (Table 2, found in the appendix to this chapter, contains a summary of many of the major cases and statutes that address this question.)

In considering parents' wrongful birth claims, the issue is what damages, if any, they ought to receive for having a child with a heritable condition whom they say they would have chosen not to bring to term. The majority of courts addressing this issue have concluded that parents may receive some sort of compensation, although they differ widely as to what the measure of damages ought to be. Looking first at economic damages, a few courts have held that the parents may recover the full cost of raising the child.[40] More frequently, courts have permitted parents to recoup the extraordinary expenses necessitated by the child's condition, but often only until the child reaches the age of majority.[41]

Courts have had more trouble deciding what to do with parents' claims for emotional injuries. Some courts have denied recovery altogether, reasoning that the parents are somehow bystanders to the child's suffering or that the mother and father did not suffer physical injury.[42] Other courts have permitted these sorts of damages, but some have required the recovery to be offset by the benefit that the parents receive from the child.[43] The diversity of responses to the claims for emotional distress is the result, in part, of continuing judicial concern that psychological injury is more likely to be trumped up and less susceptible to measurement than physical or economic harms.

Courts have had less trouble deciding what to do with the child's wrongful life claim. Since the essence of the parents' claim is the missed opportunity to avoid childbearing, most judges interpret the children's claims as assertions that they would be better off never having been born. For a variety of reasons, ranging from the metaphysical difficulty of comparing life with defects with no life at all, to judicial reluctance to say that life is ever not worth living, to views that the physician's actions harmed only the parents, most courts have simply refused to allow these children to receive damages.[44] A few courts, however, have permitted children affected by genetic disorders to recover a limited measure of damages, usually to the sum of the extraordinary costs of their care that would accrue after they reach majority.[45]

Because so much of the judicial analysis in previous cases focused on the issue of damages, it rarely mattered whether the parents said that they would have avoided procreation altogether or whether they asserted only that they were denied the opportunity to have an abortion. The only exception was in discussions of causation. Recently, however, a growing number of legislatures have stepped in to limit wrongful birth and wrongful life claims, and in some instances it makes an enormous difference exactly what choice the parents say was foreclosed to them. Although a few state legislatures have stated simply that parents and especially children cannot prevail in any cases involving allegedly inadequate genetic counseling,[46] more have denied such claims only if they are based on allegations that had the parents been adequately informed, they would have had an abortion.[47] In the latter states, parents can pursue their claims if they allege that had they been given the information at the appropriate time, they would have avoided having a child with a genetic disorder by using some of the new reproductive technologies or by not having any more children at all. This legislative approach demonstrates that the debate about abortion is much more powerful politically than is the discourse about contraception or alternative methods of procreation.

Judicial and legislative efforts to limit claims for wrongful birth and wrongful life have not gone unopposed in court. A number of litigants in recent years have argued that their due process rights were impaired by such restrictions.[48] The complainants assert, in essence, that their rights to make informed procreative choices were unduly burdened because the bans on private causes of action encouraged physicians to be negligent in warning about the risks of having a child affected by genetic disorders. Such arguments have, however, been uniformly rejected.

In summary, parents who feel that they were inappropriately denied genetic information face several hurdles if they seek to sue their health care providers. The parents bear the burden of proving that their physicians were negligent and that the deviation caused the parents to suffer damages recoverable in their state, all this in a time when state legislatures are intervening to limit such claims. Parents also run into serious problems when statutes limit the period of time in which they can sue, and they frequently find that their claims are time barred.[49] The children themselves almost never succeed in their lawsuits. Despite those difficulties, some parents do prevail and, when they do, can recover large amounts of money. This creates powerful incentive for individual practitioners to be diligent in taking genetic histories, looking for indicators of increased genetic risk, and offering reproductive genetic testing.

The Role of the Law in Abortion

In the preceding discussion of legislative, administrative, and judicial efforts to deal directly with reproductive genetic services, the current debate about abortion casts a large shadow. Tennessee, for example, specifically refuses to provide prenatal genetic testing if there is no treatment available for the affected fetus, and a number of states forbid lawsuits based on the allegation that parents were denied the opportunity to choose abortion. Analysis of the abortion statutes themselves demonstrates that they, too, can affect the availability and usefulness of genetic testing. Such an inquiry also provides more insight into the acceptance particularly of prenatal diagnosis. To this end, my focus here is on the statutes that are actually on the books. Although many of these laws have been enjoined and so have no current legal effect, the Supreme Court in *Planned Parenthood v. Casey* recently made clear that substantial, if not unlimited, state regulation may be permissible.[50]

As is true of the laws dealing directly with the availability of genetic services, it is useful to begin by looking at federal law regarding abortion, even though most of the legislation actually occurs at the state level. Since the 1970s, the United States government has refused in most instances to permit its funds to be used to pay for abortion unless the pregnancy was the result of rape or incest or unless continuing the pregnancy would threaten the life of the woman.[51] Current regulations now state explicitly that this ban applies to genetic testing funded within Maternal and Child Health Services Block Grants.[52]

The government also promulgated regulations stating that employers cannot be charged with sex discrimination if they refuse to provide "[h]ealth insurance benefits for abortion, except where the life of the mother would be endangered if the fetus were carried to term or where medical complications have arisen from an abortion . . . "[53] Employers are, however, free to provide broader benefits if they choose or if required to do so by a bargaining agreement. Thus, Congress and the administration have done much to ensure that women who seek to abort fetuses with genetic or other anomalies will have to pay for the procedures out of their own pockets.

While the impact of these congressional and administrative efforts to erect economic barriers has been far-reaching, the most profound federal influence on the law of abortion has been the elaboration in *Roe v. Wade* of limited constitutional protection of a woman's right to choose to terminate a pregnancy.[54] Before 1973, most states had restrictive statutes regarding abortion. After the decision in *Roe*, some states simply left their old statutes on the books.[55] Other states took a different approach: Some simply repealed their old laws and put nothing in their place, others enacted new laws that essentially followed the trimester approach set forth in the Supreme Court's opinion (Hood, Kavass, & Galvin, 1991). Many state legislatures, however, began to test the limits of *Roe*. Until recently, the legislatures did not assault *Roe's* basic framework directly, trying instead to attack it at the edges, passing laws, for example, requiring spousal and parental consent or notification,[56] regulating the conditions under and methods by which abortions could be performed,[57] or attempting to define viability. These efforts met with varying degrees of success in surviving constitutional scrutiny,[58] but left intact the basic notion that women could obtain abortions for any reason until the fetus reached viability.

For the most part, legislators attempted to regulate the reasons for which women could seek abortions only after fetal viability. A few states passed statutes that explicitly or implicitly permit third-trimester abortions of fetuses with serious defects,[59] but most that addressed the issue allow late abortions only if continuing the pregnancy would threaten the life or health of the woman.[60] Although one state sought to restrict certain abortions prior to viability,[61] the others that considered decisions made during this period took a more permissive stance, mentioning the presence of defects in the fetus only as a factor to be considered, and usually by the physician.[62] (The language of the statutes that address the legal implications of finding defects in the fetus for abortion decisions are summarized in table 3 of this chapter's appendix.) The result of the relative silence on the federal and state level about selective abortion has been that women can legally abort fetuses with defects before viability and sometimes thereafter.

However, beginning early in the 1980s and culminating in *Webster v. Reproductive Health Services*,[63] a growing number of the justices on the Supreme Court expressed dissatisfaction with *Roe v. Wade* and essentially invited the states to pursue a more frontal assault on the earlier opinion. In response to this judicial rhetoric, as well as to growing political pressure, legislators began to devote much more attention to abortion, resulting in a spate of new laws. A few legislatures accepted the invitation of the discontented justices and enacted very restrictive statutes that fly in the face of *Roe*. Utah, for example, passed a law that would permit abortion only if the pregnancy threatened the life of the woman or was the result of rape or incest, or if the fetus was diagnosed with grave defects.[64] Louisiana's new law is even more restrictive, allowing abortion only if the pregnancy was caused by rape or incest or threatens the woman's life.[65] Guam's statute permits abortion only when the pregnancy is ectopic or when two physicians independently agree that "there is a substantial risk that continuance of the pregnancy would endanger the life of the mother or would gravely impair the health of the mother."[66] Notably, the latter two statutes contain no provision for selective abortion of fetuses with anomalies.

For now, the validity of these restrictions must be assessed in the light of the Supreme Court's recent opinion in *Planned Parenthood v. Casey*.[67] In that case, the Court held that while legislatures may regulate abortions prior to viability, they may not place undue burdens in the way of a woman's right to choose. Because requirements that married women notify their spouses and that minors notify both their parents[68] have been held to be undue burdens, the scope of permissible regulation, while quite broad, is not unlimited. Indeed, Louisiana's and Guam's statutes have already been struck down.[69] A district court in Utah, however, in an opinion handed down days before *Casey*, upheld the Utah statute, rejecting among other things an argument that the provision that abortions be permitted only when the fetus suffered from grave defects was unconstitutionally vague.[70] In the unlikely event that the district court's ruling upholding limitations on abortions of fetuses with defects survives appeal, it would open the door to other states that wish to limit women's ability to decide to abort fetuses with anomalies or other genetic disorders. Women who live in states that adopt laws as restrictive as Utah's may be forced to travel to another more permissive state if they seek an abortion after prenatal testing detects a problem in the developing fetus. While this additional hurdle is one that some women will not be able to surmount, other courts have found restrictions that force women to undertake burdensome travel not to be undue.[71]

The United States Constitution is not the only protection available to women opposing state legislatures' efforts to restrict access to abortion. Women increasingly assert, with varying degrees of success, that their state constitutions protect the right to choose,[72] and the new Congress may well enact a federal statute guaranteeing some sort of access.[73] But unless Congress and state courts step in, many women face the prospect that their state governments will curtail their ability to choose to abort a fetus with defects.

Even assuming that women retain some rights to choose abortion, many women already confront substantial economic barriers to such choices that the states have done little to address. A few states have chosen to provide public funding for selective abortion, often hiding such decisions in funding bills that do not make it into the statute books where they would be readily accessible for public scrutiny. (The language of these funding provisions is summarized in table 4 of this chapter's appendix.) Most states, however, do not permit their medical assistance funds to be used for this purpose, which is hardly surprising in the light of the federal restrictions.

Fourteen legislatures also accepted the invitation of the Title VII regulations to enact laws permitting private insurers to exclude coverage for most abortions except when the pregnancy threatens the life of the woman or when complications have arisen from an earlier abortion.[74] While most of those statutes do allow insurers to offer these benefits if they choose, not a single state requires insurers to pay for abortions of fetuses with defects. Efforts are now underway to ascertain what insurers are actually doing within these legal guidelines.[75] Many privately insured women are probably covered for testing and abortion since, from the insurer's perspective, those procedures may often be cost-effective when compared to the costliness of long term care for a child with a serious genetic disease. Indeed, what some women may need more than coverage is protection from insurers' efforts to pressure them into aborting fetuses who are at risk for or who are determined to have a genetic disorder (Karjala, 1992).

Regardless of the context of private insurance, the result of most of the statutes regarding abortion is that many poor women cannot use prenatal diagnosis, even if it is offered by the state or some other party, because they cannot afford the abortion that they might want should the fetus be found to have a defect. Moreover, all women face the threat that the Supreme Court will not recognize a woman's right to abort a fetus with genetic defects when the Court is directly confronted with the question. Were this admittedly unlikely scenario to occur and were states to act aggressively to restrict selective abortion while Congress remained silent, prenatal diagnosis would have little place, at least until gene therapy or other therapeutic interventions become available.

Governmental Response to Reproductive Genetic Testing—Lacunae and Ambivalence

It would be unrealistic to expect all states to have fully developed responses to technologies as new as reproductive genetic testing. Governments simply do not move that quickly. But the lack of well thought out programs is probably the result of more than mere reluctance to deal with technical matters or the press of other problems. For as noted at the outset, the inextricable linkage between reproductive genetic testing and alternative methods of procreation, contraception, and abortion raises profound and controversial issues.

The existence of such deeply divided beliefs has meant that many legislators passed laws not always consistent with one another. Examples of such inconsistencies abound. Tennessee passed a law in 1985 forbidding the use of public funds for prenatal diagnosis of conditions for which there are no effective therapy, saying that abortion was against public policy.[76] Since 1989, however, that same legislature has provided public funds for abortions of fetuses "medically determined to have severe physical deformities or abnormalities or severe mental retardation."[77]

Louisiana established regional genetics clinics for its citizens[78] and later passed the first statute in the continental United States since *Roe v. Wade* to forbid the abortion of fetuses affected with genetic disorders.[79] Missouri will pay for "genetic diagnostic evaluations, treatment, counseling, and follow-up for families with or at high risk for a genetic disease,"[80] language that appears to include prenatal diagnosis, but forbids referral for abortion unless the life of the woman is threatened. That state also enacted a statute barring recovery for claims by parents alleging that they were denied genetic information that would have led them to choose abortion.[81] The government of North Carolina provides an extensive set of genetic services to its citizens.[82] Its highest court, however, held that neither parents nor children can receive compensation when the parents were inappropriately denied genetic information.[83] A similar set of laws providing services[84] but barring suits for wrongful birth and wrongful life[85] were enacted by Colorado's legislature.

At the other end of the spectrum, the New Jersey courts provide among the broadest recovery for wrongful birth and wrongful life claims seen in this country.[86] That state's legislature, by contrast, has done almost nothing to provide genetic services to its citizens.[87]

Some of those laws can be reconciled with each other at least on a formal level, usually on the ground that preconception testing is more acceptable than that occurring after pregnancy has begun because of the more obvious possibility of abortion in the latter case. Thus a state could offer carrier screening while declining to provide prenatal diagnosis. Even so, it is hard to understand why a state would make available genetic testing and then deny private rights of action to their citizens when individual practitioners fail to provide the same services.

Particularly in the light of the number of laws that have been enacted, it is remarkable how infrequently governmental bodies have created comprehensive sets of services and protections. Far more frequently, the legislators established programs in little more than a sentence despite their far-reaching implications. Only a handful of legislatures took a broad look at the potential needs or desires of their citizens. Few regulate the genetic testing techniques to ensure that testing is actually being done accurately.[88] Perhaps legislators are relying upon the litigation about wrongful birth and wrongful life, the efforts of private groups, and the Federal Clinical Laboratory Improvement Act[89] to elaborate appropriate standards of care even though such mechanisms are not likely to be fully effective. These technologies are often expensive, yet only a small number of states have acted to ensure that adequate funding is available to those who wish to receive testing and counseling.[90]

The lawmakers have said correspondingly little about abortions of fetuses with genetic disorders. Their silence may have been the result, until recently, of a sense that there was little reason to say anything because the law was clear. Now that the law is open to question, legislators from both ends of the political spectrum may be reluctant to address the subject of genetically indicated abortions. Perhaps some lawmakers who generally oppose choice are ambivalent when the fetus has serious defects. More likely, those who favor choice fear the consequences of opening the topic for discussion at all.

Legislators have said nothing about the use of alternative methods of procreation such as artificial insemination by donor and egg donation as possible methods to avoid having children with genetic disorders. This lack of activity is not particularly surprising since regulation of the new reproductive technologies has been an area that legislatures have hesitated to confront. Indeed, only one state requires physicians to obtain a genetic history from sperm donors, and that state only suggests genetic testing.[91] Their silence, nonetheless, reveals yet another way in which lawmakers have failed to ensure that families have options in the face of information indicating that they may produce children with genetic disorders.

Finally, in addition to the inconsistencies and gaps within the policies of individual states, it is also obvious that the variation among the public policies of different states is enormous. California, which has worked on many levels to increase access to

reproductive genetic testing, has radically different policies
from Louisiana, which has sought to ban abortion altogether in
most situations. Taken as a whole, the frequency with which
individual states have adopted conflicting or perfunctory policies, or no policies at all, and the wide array of approaches taken
by the different states demonstrate that there is no consensus on
the role of reproductive genetic testing.

Conclusion

The law affects reproductive genetic testing in a host of ways.
Legislators, congresspeople, and administrators have sought
both to provide and to limit access to genetic testing. When the
government attempts to ensure access, it often provides services
itself, and less frequently requires third-party payers to provide
coverage. In those efforts, however, it is truly remarkable how
rarely the links between reproductive genetic testing, contraception, abortion, alternative methods of procreation, and feelings of discomfort about the "new genetics" have actually been
acknowledged. The implications have been more explicitly recognized when legislatures put barriers in the way of individuals'
desires to obtain reproductive genetic testing. But no matter
what form the discussion takes, the implications for women of
this sort of testing are rarely considered.

The most powerful force driving the use of these technologies is not the direct interventions of governments to ensure
access, rather it is the actions of individual litigants who bear a
child affected with a genetic disorder and then sue health care
providers and institutions. That genetic testing would be shaped
more by lawsuits than by legislation is hardly surprising since
litigants are not constrained by the same political pressures and
public rhetoric that lawmakers face. The individuals who have
sued physicians and health care institutions have alleged that
they were entitled to information that can be revealed by reproductive genetic testing. The sense that those people were
wronged by being denied this information has been supported,
albeit to varying degrees, by the courts and only partially undermined by legislative efforts to limit such suits.

The wealth of articles and books in the genetics literature as well as informal conversations with geneticists and genetic counselors suggest that the private lawsuits are viewed as powerful incentives for encouraging the use of genetic testing. Indeed providers seem to have been driven, by their fear of liability, to expand the care they deliver. This more sophisticated level of practice has elevated the standard of care, thereby, almost ironically, increasing individual practitioners' potential exposure to claims that they failed to provide appropriate care.

One might argue that these cases demonstrate that women very much want reproductive genetic testing. But before one accepts this hypothesis too readily, one must recognize that individuals' reasons for claiming can be quite complex, ranging from anger at a physician's lack of communication skills or the desire for genetic information, to pressure from others or the simple need for money (Hickson, Clayton, Githens, & Sloan, 1992; Sloan et al., 1993). Thus, more scrutiny of the events that led families to pursue claims for wrongful birth and wrongful life is necessary. Even if the people who sued did feel that they were wronged by being denied access to genetic information, it is also possible that they would have been troubled by their options had the information been provided. And there is no reason to think that most people hold the same views about the desirability of reproductive genetic testing as those who filed claims.

The result of legislative and administrative actions and private litigation is a two-tiered system. People who are poor have some access to genetic services, limited in many instances by debate and ambivalence within the political arena. Their ability to obtain access via court, seeking damages for wrongful birth or wrongful life, is limited because they cannot prove causation should they not have been able to pay for the services they say they were denied. Individuals who can pay, by contrast, have greater access to genetic testing—access facilitated by patterns of medical practice driven by the pressures of litigation and by a wish for cost-efficiency by insurers.

The gap between the two levels of service may narrow in the future. The poor may be given greater access, perhaps for unspoken eugenic reasons or perhaps due to greater political activism by those who are pro-choice or who view procreative decision-making as a personal matter. An alternative scenario is that legislatures will limit or bar the claims of individuals who do not receive genetic information, thereby limiting the incentives of practitioners to provide genetic testing. Another more distant possibility is that legislatures will successfully limit the use of abortion in cases where fetuses are determined to have genetic or other disorders.

Given the dramatic increases in genetic knowledge, it seems likely legislatures will continue to address reproductive genetic testing. But if inconsistent and incomplete policies are to be avoided, the implications of this technology for contraception, abortion, and alternative methods of procreation, and ultimately for the ways in which we regard others must be confronted directly. It will also be necessary to decide what interests ought appropriately to be considered and what weight those interests should be given. The role of promoting reproductive genetic testing for eugenic purposes and for avoiding burdens on the public fisc must be explicitly addressed. A major challenge will be to ensure that the various views of women are heard in the debate.

ACKNOWLEDGMENTS

I would like to thank Jay Clayton and Karen Rothenberg for their insightful comments on earlier drafts, Dorris Baker and Danette Watkins for their assistance with preparation of the manuscript and tables, Alvina Ma for her assistance with research, and the staff of the Vanderbilt Law School Library for their research support.

NOTES

1. See Reilly (1991); *Buck v. Bell*, 274 U.S. 200 (1927); and *In re* Sterilization of Moore, 221 S.E.2d 307 (N.C. 1976).
2. See Reilly (1987); Pub. L. No. 94–278, §§ 401–403, 90 Stat. 407, codified at 42 U.S.C. §§ 300b-300b-3; H. Rep. No, 94–498, 94th Cong., 2d Sess., reprinted in 1976 U.S.C.C.A.N. 709; and H. Conf. Rep. 94–1005, 94th Cong., 2d Sess. reprinted in 1976 U.S.C.C.A.N. 742.
3. 42 U.S.C.A. § 701 & 702 (1992).
4. 42 C.F.R. §§ 51f.101–110.
5. Removal of obsolete regulations on hemophilia treatment centers and genetic disease testing and counseling programs, 53 Fed. Reg. 27859 (1988).
6. 42 C.F.R. § 51a.7 (1991).
7. 42 U.S.C.A. § 300b-1 (1992).
8. 42 U.S.C.A. § 300b-4 (1992).

9. 38 U.S.C.A. § 662 (1992) (preventive health care services pilot program for some veterans).

10. 32 C.F.R. § 199.4(e)(3)(ii) (1991).

11. 32 C.F.R. § 199.4(e)(2) (1991).

12. 32 C.F.R. § 728.31(d)(9) (1991); 32 C.F.R. § 728.71(b)(1) (1991).

13. Ala. Code §§ 22–10A-1-3 (1991) (genetics program); Cal. Health & Safety Code §§ 150–156.3 (1991) (Hereditary Diseases Act and prenatal diagnosis); Cal. Health & Safety Code § 309.5 (1991) (genetic disease fund); Md. Pub. Health Code Ann. §§ 13-101-111 (1991) (hereditary and congenital disorders program); Mass. Gen. Laws Ann. ch. 76, § 15B (1991) (genetic screening); Mo. Ann. Stat. §§ 191.300-.380 (1991) (genetics and metabolic disease programs); N.C. Gen. Stat. § 95–28.1 (1991) (anti-discrimination; sickle-cell trait or hemoglobin C trait); Ohio Rev. Code Ann. § 3701.502 (1989) (genetics program); Tex. Health & Safety Code Ann. §§ 134.001-.007 (1991) (Interagency Council for Genetic Services).

14. Ga. Code Ann. § 31-12-5 (1991) (medical genetics services); Minn. Stat. Ann. § 144.91 (1991) (genetics program); Minn. Stat. Ann. § 144.925 (1991) (genetic counseling as part of family planning); N.Y. Pub. Health Law §§ 2730–2733 (1991) (Birth Defects Institute); Utah Code Ann. § 26-5-2 (1990) (genetics program as part of effort to prevent chronic disease).

15. Fla. Stat. Ann. § 393.064 (1991) (developmental disabilities of genetic origin); N.C. Gen. Stat. § 95–28.1 (1991) (anti-discrimination; sickle-cell trait or hemoglobin C trait); P.R. Laws Ann. § 3156 (1990) (genetic counseling associated with newborn screening).

16. La. Admin. Code §§ 6501–3, 6901–3 (1987) (genetics program and advisory committee).

17. Ala. Code §§ 22–10A-1-3 (1991) (genetics program); Cal. Health & Safety Code §§ 150–156.3 (1991) (Hereditary Diseases Act and prenatal diagnosis); Hawaii Rev. Stat. § 321–331 (1990) (prenatal diagnosis); Me. Rev. Stat. Ann. tit. 22, § 1533 (1989) (genetics program); 1991 Nev. Stat. 622 (genetics program, including prenatal diagnosis), codified at Nev. Rev. Stat. Ann. §§ 396.521-.527 (1991); Or. Rev. Stat. §§ 352.055-.058 (1991) (genetics program and prenatal diagnosis); Utah Code Ann. § 26-10-1 (1990) (suggesting that some prenatal diagnosis may be provided under maternal/child health); Wash. Rev. Code Ann. §§ 70.83B.010-.900 (1990) (prenatal diagnosis).

18. 77 Ill. Admin. Code § 630.30 (1985) (MCH project to cover genetic screening and prenatal diagnosis); Md. Admin. Code tit. 10, §§ 39.02.01-.10, 39.03.01-.06, 52.01.01-.06 (genetics programs and MSAFP); Ohio Admin. Code §§ 5101:3-4-07&08 (1989) (genetics within family planning and obstetrical services).

19. 1991 Minn. Ch. Laws 33, § 36 (some insurance benefits to cover prenatal diagnosis), to be codified at Minn. Stat. Ann. ch. 62K; Minn. R. § 9505.0235 (1991) (Medicaid will pay for ultrasound and laboratory tests to detect fetal abnormalities); Mo. Ann. Stat. §§ 191.300-.380 (1991) (genetics and metabolic disease programs).

20. Tenn. Code Ann. § 68-5-504(a) (1991).

21. 1991 Pa. Law 40-A & 1992 Pa. Law 34A (establishing program for Tay-Sachs at Jefferson Medical College).
22. La. Rev. Stat. Ann. § 28:381(16) (1991) (genetic counseling for families of mentally retarded or developmentally disabled); Mich. Comp. Laws Ann. §§ 333.5401-.5439 (1991) (chronic disease program, which includes genetics).
23. Cal. Civ. Code § 4201.5 (1991) (brochure to marriage applicants); Ill. Ann. Stat. ch. 127, ¶ 55.55 (1991) (brochure for applicants for marriage license); N.Y. Pub. Health Law §§ 2730–2733 (1991) (Birth Defects Institute); Va. Code §§ 32.1–68&69 (1990) (genetics program).
24. Kan. Stat. Ann. §§ 65–1,105–1,106 (1990) (sickle-cell testing including advising parents of new school entrants of possibility of testing).
25. Cal. Health & Safety Code §1367.7 (1991) (health care service plan coverage of prenatal diagnosis); Cal. Ins. Code § 10123.9 (1991) (group policy coverage of prenatal diagnosis); Cal. Ins. Code § 11512.18 (1991) (nonprofit hospital service plan coverage of prenatal diagnosis); 1991 Minn. Ch. Laws 33, § 36 (some insurance benefits to cover prenatal diagnosis), to be codified at Minn. Stat. Ann. ch. 62K; Wash. Rev. Code Ann. § 48.21.244 (1990) (group disability to pay for prenatal diagnosis); Wash. Rev. Code Ann. § 48.44.344 (1990) (group health care services contract to cover prenatal diagnosis); Wash. Rev. Code Ann. § 48.46.375 (1990) (HMOs to cover prenatal diagnosis).
26. La. Rev. Stat. Ann. § 215.8 (1991) (insurance for cleft lip/palate, if provided, must include genetic counseling).
27. 77 Ill. Admin. Code § 630.30 (1985) (MCH project to cover genetic screening and prenatal diagnosis); Minn. Stat. Ann. § 144.925 (1991) (genetic counseling as part of family planning); Ohio Admin. Code §§ 5101:3-4-07&08 (1989) (genetics within family planning and obstetrical services); Wis. Admin. Code § HSS 107.21 (1986) (family planning includes range of services including prenatal diagnosis).
28. 53 Fed. Reg. 2922–2946 (1988), codified at 42 C.F.R. §§ 59.2–59.10.
29. 500 U.S. 173 (1991).
30. *Robak v. U.S.*, 658 F.2d 471 (7th Cir. 1981) (Alabama law).
31. *Howard v. Lecher*, 366 N.E.2d 64 (NY 1977) (alleging failure to recognize risk that parents who are Ashkenazi Jews may have child with Tay-Sachs disease).
32. *Atlanta Obstet. Gynecol. Group v. Abelson*, 398 S.E.2d 557 (Ga. 1990) (advanced maternal age); *Berman v. Allan*, 404 A.2d 8 (N.J. 1979) (advanced maternal age); *Becker v. Schwartz*, 386 N.E.2d 64 (N.Y. 1977) (advanced maternal age).
33. *Turpin v. Sortini*, 643 P.2d 954 (Cal. 1982) (congenital deafness); *Moores v. Lucas*, 405 So.2d 1022 (Fla. Ct. App. 1981) (Larsen's syndrome); *Schroeder v. Perkel*, 432 A.2d 834 (N.J. 1981) (cystic fibrosis); *Park v. Chessin*, 400 N.Y.S.2d 110 (App. Div. 1977), modified on appeal sub nom., *Becker v. Schwartz*, 386 N.E.2d 807 (N.Y. 1978) (polycystic kidney disease).
34. *Curlender v. Bio-Science Laboratories*, 165 Cal. Rptr. 477 (Cal. App. 1980).
35. *Robak v. U.S.*, 658 F.2d 471 (7th Cir. 1981) (Alabama law).

36. *Keselman v. Kingsboro Med. Grp.*, 548 N.Y.S.2d 287, 288 (App. Div. 1989), app dism'd without opinion sub nom.; *Keselman v. Flatbush Med. Grp.*, 559 N.E.2d 1288 (N.Y. 1990).
37. *Roe v. Wade*, 410 U.S. 113 (1973).
38. *Gleitman v. Cosgrove*, 227 A.2d 689 (N.J. 1967); *Hummel v. Reiss*, 608 A.2d 1341 (N.J. 1992) (negligence occurred before 1973).
39. *Elliot v. Brown*, 361 So.2d 546 (Ala. 1978).
40. *Robak v. U.S.*, 658 F.2d 471 (7th Cir. 1981) (Alabama law); *Gallagher v. Duke Univ.*, 852 F.2d 773 (4th Cir. 1988) (North Carolina law); *Speck v. Finegold*, 439 A.2d 110 (Pa. 1981).
41. *Becker v. Schwartz*, 386 N.E.2d 64 (N.Y. 1977) (advanced maternal age); *Schroeder v. Perkel*, 432 A.2d 834 (N.J. 1981) (cystic fibrosis); *Walker v. Mart*, 790 P.2d 735 (Ariz. 1990); Colo. Rev. Stat. § 13-64-502 (1991); *Ochs v. Borelli*, 445 A.2d 883 (Conn. 1982); *Donnelly v. Candlewood Obstet-Gynecol. Assoc.*, No. 30 20 96, 1992 Conn. Super. LEXIS 1682 (June 8, 1992); *Haymon v. Wilkerson*, 535 A.2d 880 (D.C. App. 1987); *Garrison v. Medical Center of Del.*, 581 A.2d 288 (Del. 1990); *Fassoulas v. Ramey*, 450 So.2d 984 (Fla. 1984); *Blake v. Cruz*, 698 P.2d 315 (Idaho 1984); *Sieminiec v. Lutheran Gen. Hosp.*, 512 N.E.2d 691 (Ill. 1987); *Arche v. U.S.*, 798 P.2d 477 (Kan. 1990); *Pines v. Moreno*, 569 So.2d 203 (La. App. 1990); Me. Rev. Stat. Ann. tit. 24, § 2931 (1989); *Viccaro v. Milunsky*, 551 N.E.2d 8 (Mass. 1990); *Proffit v. Bartolo*, 412 N.W.2d 232 (Mich. App. 1987); *Smith v. Cote*, 513 A.2d 341 (N.H. 1986); *Bani-Esraili v. Lerman*, 505 N.E.2d 947 (N.Y. 1987); *Gallagher v. Duke Univ.*, 852 F.2d 773 (4th Cir. 1988) (North Carolina law); *Stribling v. deQuevedo*, 432 A.2d 239 (Pa. Super. 1980); *Naccash v. Burger*, 290 S.E.2d 825 (Va. 1982); *Harbeson v. Parke-Davis*, 656 P.2d 483 (Wash. 1983); *Harbeson v. Parke-Davis*, 746 F.2d 517 (9th Cir. 1984) (Washington law); *James G. v. Caserta*, 332 S.E.2d 872 (W. Va. 1985); *Dumer v. St. Michaels Hosp.*, 233 N.W. 2d 372 (Wis. 1975).
42. *Howard v. Lecher*, 366 N.E.2d 64 (NY 1977) (alleging failure to recognize risk that parents who are Ashkenazi Jews may have child with Tay-Sachs disease); *Becker v. Schwartz*, 386 N.E.2d 64 (N.Y. 1977) (advanced maternal age); *Turpin v. Sortini*, 643 P.2d 954 (Cal. 1982); *Garrison v. Medical Center of Del.*, 581 A.2d 288 (Del. 1990); *Sieminiec v. Lutheran Gen. Hosp.*, 512 N.E.2d 691 (Ill. 1987); *Arche v. U.S.*, 798 P.2d 477 (Kan. 1990).
43. *Blake v. Cruz*, 698 P.2d 315 (Idaho 1984); *Viccaro v. Milunsky*, 551 N.E.2d 8 (Mass. 1990); *Phillips v. U.S.*, 575 F. Supp. 1309 (D.S.C. 1983).
44. *Becker v. Schwartz*, 386 N.E.2d 64 (N.Y. 1977) (advanced maternal age); *Moores v. Lucas*, 405 So.2d 1022 (Fla. Ct. App. 1981) (Larsen's syndrome); *Elliot v. Brown*, 361 So.2d 546 (Ala. 1978); *Walker v. Mart*, 790 P.2d 735 (Ariz. 1990); *Andalon v. Super Ct.*, 208 Cal. Rptr. 899 (Cal. App. 1984); *Lininger v. Eisenbaum*, 764 P.2d 1202 (Colo. 1988); *Garrison v. Medical Center of Del.*, 581 A.2d 288 (Del. 1990); *Lloyd v. North Broward Hosp. Dist.*, 570 So.2d 984 (Fla. App. 1990); *Blake v. Cruz*, 698 P.2d 315 (Idaho 1984); *Sieminiec v. Lutheran Gen.*

Hosp., 512 N.E.2d 691 (Ill. 1987); *Goldberg v. Ruskin*, 499 N.E.2d 406 (Ill. 1986); *Cowe v. Forum Grp.*, 575 N.E.2d 630 (Ind. 1991); *Bruggeman v. Schimke*, 718 P.2d 635 (Kan. 1986); *Viccaro v. Milunsky*, 551 N.E.2d 8 (Mass. 1990); *Eisbrenner v. Stanley*, 308 N.W.2d 209 (Mich. App. 1981); *Wilson v. Kuenzi*, 751 S.W.2d 741 (Mo. 1988); *Smith v. Cote*, 513 A.2d 341 (N.H. 1986); *Alquijay v. St. Luke's-Roosevelt Hosp. Ctr.*, 473 N.E.2d 244 (N.Y. 1984); *Azzolino v. Dingfelder*, 337 S.E.2d 528 (N.C. 1985), cert. denied, 479 U.S. 835 (1986); *Ellis v. Sherman*, 515 A.2d 1327 (Pa. 1986); *Stribling v. deQuevedo*, 432 A.2d 239 (Pa. Super. 1980); *Phillips v. U.S.*, 508 F. Supp. 537 (D.S.C. 1980); *Nelson v. Krusen*, 678 S.W.2d 918 (Tex. 1984); *James G. v. Caserta*, 332 S.E.2d 872 (W. Va. 1985); *Dumer v. St. Michaels Hosp.*, 233 N.W. 2d 372 (Wis. 1975).

45. *Turpin v. Sortini*, 643 P.2d 954 (Cal. 1982) (congenital deafness); *Pines v. Moreno*, 569 So.2d 203 (La. App. 1990); *Procanik v. Cillo*, 478 A.2d 755 (N.J. 1984); *Harbeson v. Parke-Davis*, 656 P.2d 483 (Wash. 1983); *Harbeson v. Parke-Davis*, 746 F.2d 517 (9th Cir. 1984) (Washington law).

46. Colo. Rev. State. § 13-64-502 (1991); Me. Rev. Stat. Ann. tit. 24, § 2931 (1989); Pa. Stat. Ann. tit. 42, § 8305 (1991); S. Dak. Codified Laws Ann. §§ 21-55-1 & -2 (1991).

47. Idaho Code § 5-334 (1991); Ind. Code Ann. § 34-1-1-11 (1991); Minn. Stat. Ann. § 145.424 (1991); Mo. Ann. Stat. § 188.130 (1991); Utah Code Ann. § 78-11-24 (1990).

48. *Campbell v. U.S.*, 962 F.2d 1579 (11th Cir. 1992) (Georgia law); *Spires v. Kim*, 416 S.E.2d 780 (Ga. App. 1992); *Edmonds v. Western Pennsylvania Hosp. Radiology Assoc.*, 607 A.2d 1083 (Pa. Super. 1992).

49. *Dorlin v. Providence Hosp.*, 325 N.W.2d 600 (Mich. App. 1982); *Procanik v. Cillo*, 478 A.2d 755 (N.J. 1984); *Alquijay v. St. Luke's-Roosevelt Hosp. Ctr.*, 473 N.E.2d 244 (N.Y. 1984); *Brubaker v. Cavanaugh*, 741 F.2d 318 (10th Cir. 1984) (Kansas law); *Payne v. Myers*, 743 P.2d 186 (Utah 1987).

50. *Planned Parenthood of Southeastern Pennsylvania v. Casey*, 112 S.Ct. 2791 (1992).

51. 42 U.S.C.A. § 300a-6 (1991) (no funds to programs in which abortion used as method for family planning); 28 C.F.R. §551.23(b) (1990) (prison inmates); 42 C.F.R. § 36.54 (1990) (Indian Health Services; mentions only life of the woman); 42 C.F.R. §§ 50.304, 50.306 (1990) (Public Health Service).

52. 42 C.F.R. § 51a.7 (1991).

53. 29 C.F.R. § 1604.10 (1991) (explicating Title VII).

54. *Roe v. Wade*, 410 U.S. 113 (1973).

55. N.H. Rev. Stat. Ann. §§ 585:12-14 (1991).

56. Ill. Rev. Stat. Ch. 110, ¶ 11-107. 1 (1987); Ala. Code §§ 26-21-1-8 (1988); Minn. Stat. § 144.343 (1988); Ohio Rev. Code Ann. §§ 2151.85, 2505.073, 2919.12 (1989); Tenn. Code Ann. §§ 37-10-301-307 (1988).

57. Conn. Gen. Stat. § 19a-116 (1988); Tex. Rev. Civ. Stat. Ann. art 4512.8 (1989).

58. *Planned Parenthood of Central Missouri v. Danforth*, 428 U.S. 52 (1976); *Colautti v. Franklin*, 439 U.S. 379 (1979); *Thornburgh v. American Coll. Obstet. Gynecol.*, 476 U.S. 747 (1986).
59. Idaho Code § 18–608 (1991); Kan. Stat. Ann. § 21–3407 (1991); Md. Pub. Health Code Ann. § 20–208 (1991); N.H. Rev. Stat. Ann. § 585.13 (1991); Pa. Cons. Stat. Ann. tit. 18, § 3204 (1991); Tex. Rev. Civ. Stat. Ann. art 44956 (1991); 1991 Utah Laws ch. 2, codified at Utah Code Ann. §§ 76-7-301-317.1 (1992).
60. Ariz. Rev. Stat. Ann. § 36–2301.01 (1991); Ark. Stat. Ann. § 20-16-705 (1991); Conn. Gen. Stat. Ann. § 19a-602 (1990); Fla. Stat. § 390.001(2) (1991); Ga. Code Ann. § 16-12-141(d) (1991); Ill. Rev. Stat. ch. 38, ¶ 81–25 (1989); Ind. Code Ann. § 35-1-58.5–2 (3) (1990); Ky. Rev. Stat. Ann. § 311.780 (1991); 1991 La. Act 2, codified at La. Rev. Stat. Ann. § 14.87 (1992); 22 Me. Rev. Stat. Ann. § 1598.4 (1991); Mass. Gen. Laws Ann. ch. 112, § 12M (1991); Minn. Stat. § 145.412. subd. 3 (1991); Mont. Code Ann. § 50-20-109(1)(c) (1991); Neb. Rev. Stat. § 28–329 (1988); Nev. Rev. Stat. Ann. § 442.250.1.(c) (1990); N.C. Gen. Stat. § 14–45.1(b) (1990); N.D. Cent. Code § 14–02.1–04.3 (1991); Okla. Stat. tit. 63, § 1–732 (1990); 18 Pa. Cons. Stat. Ann. § 3211 (1992); S.C. Code Ann. § 44-41-20(c) (Law. Co-op. 1990); Tenn. Code Ann. § 39-15-201(c)(3) (1991); Va. Code Ann. § 18.2–74 (1991); Wis. Stat. § 940.15(3) (1989–90); Wyo. Stat. § 35-6-102 (1991).
61. Pa. Cons. Stat. Ann. tit. 18, § 3204 (1991).
62. Del. Code Ann. tit. 24, § 1790 (1991); Idaho Code § 18–608 (1991); Kan. Stat. Ann. § 21–3407 (1991); Md. Pub. Health Code Ann. § 20–208 (1991); N.H. Rev. Stat. Ann. § 585.13 (1991); Tex. Rev. Civ. Stat. Ann. art 44956 (1991).
63. 492 U.S. 490 (1989).
64. 1991 Utah Laws ch. 2, codified at Utah Code Ann. §§ 76-7-301-317.1 (1992).
65. 1991 La. Act 2, codified at La. Rev. Stat. Ann. § 14.87 (1992).
66. Guam Pub. L. No. 20–134, codified at Guam Code Ann. §§ 31.20–31.23.
67. *Planned Parenthood of Southeastern Pennsylvania v. Casey*, 112 S.Ct. 2791 (1992).
68. *Hodgson v. Minnesota*, 110 S.Ct. 2926 (1990).
69. *Sojourner T. v. Edwards*, 974 F.2d 27 (5th Cir. 1992); *Guam Soc'y Obstet Gynecol v. Ada*, No. 90–16706, 1992 U.S. App. LEXIS 13490 (9th Cir. 1992).
70. *Jane L. v. Bangerter*, 794 F. Supp. 1537 (D. Utah 1992).
71. *Planned Parenthood of Southeastern Pennsylvania v. Casey*, 112 S.Ct. 2791 (1992); *Barnes v. Moore*, 970 F.2d 12 (5th Cir.), cert. denied, 61 U.S.L.W. 3418 (1992).
72. *Comm. to Defend Reproductive Rights v. Myers*, 625 P.2d 779 (Cal. 1981); *In re* T.W., No. 74,143, 1989 Fla. LEXIS 1226 (Fla. 1989); *Moe v. Secretary Admin. Fin.*, 417 N.E.2d 387 (Mass. 1981); *Right to Choose v. Byrne*, 450 A.2d 925 (N.J. 1982).
73. *Freedom of Choice Act of 1992*, S. 25, 102d Cong. 2d Sess. (1991).

74. Idaho Code §§ 41–2142, 2210A, 3439, & 3934 (1991); Ill. Rev. Stat. Ann. chs. 73 ¶ 1308, 127 ¶¶ 526, 526.1 (1991); 1992 Ill. Pub. Act 1164, § 1 (13); Iowa Code §§ 601A.6 & .13 (1989); Ky. Rev. Stat. Ann. §§ 304.18–120 & .32–310 (1991); Minn. Stat. §§ 62A.041, D.02, D.20, & D.22 (1991); Mo. Rev. Stat. § 376.805 (1990); 1991 Mont. Laws ch. 798 § 31(xii); Neb. Rev. Stat. § 44–1615.01 (1990); N.D. Cent. Code § 14–02.3–03 (1991); Ohio Rev. Code Ann. § 4112.01 (1991); 18 Pa. Cons. Stat. § 3215(E) (1989); 31 Pa. Admin. Code § 89.77(a)(ii) (1989); R.I. Gen. Laws §§ 27-18-28 & 36-12-2.1 (1990); S.C. Code Ann. § 1-13-30 (Law. Co-op. 1990).

75. Moseley R. "Insurance Implications of a Complete Genome Map," 1 R01 HG 00402–01.

76. Tenn. Code Ann. § 68-5-504(a) (1991).

77. 1992 Tenn. Pub. Act. 1018, § 10, Item 4(3).

78. Kan. Stat. Ann. §§ 65–1,105–1,106 (1990) (sickle-cell testing including advising parents of new school entrants of possibility of testing).

79. 1991 La. Act 2, codified at La. Rev. Stat. Ann. § 14.87 (1992).

80. Mo. Ann. Stat. § 191.320 (1991).

81. Mo. Ann. Stat. § 188.130 (1991).

82. N.C. Admin. Code tit. 15A, §§ 21H.0301-.0313 (1991) (genetics program).

83. *Azzolino v. Dingfelder*, 337 S.E.2d 528 (N.C. 1985), cert. denied, 479 U.S. 835 (1986).

84. Colo. Rev. Stat. §§ 25-4-1001-1006 (1991) (Newborn Screening and Genetic Counseling and Education Act).

85. Colo. Rev. State. § 13-64-502 (1991).

86. *Berman v. Allan*, 404 A.2d 8 (N.J. 1979) (advanced maternal age); *Schroeder v. Perkel*, 432 A.2d 834 (N.J. 1981) (cystic fibrosis); *Procanik v. Cillo*, 478 A.2d 755 (N.J. 1984).

87. N.J. Stat. Ann. §§ 26:5B-1-4 (1991) (hereditary disorders); N.J. Stat. Ann. § 37:1–27 (1991) (brochures to applicants for marriage licenses).

88. Cal. Health & Safety Code §§ 150–156.3 (1991) (Hereditary Diseases Act and prenatal diagnosis); Hawaii Rev. Stat. § 321–331 (1990) (prenatal diagnosis); Iowa Code Ann. §§ 136A.1–7 (1991) (Birth Defects Institute); Md. Pub. Health Code Ann. §§ 13-101-111 (1991) (hereditary and congenital disorders program); Mo. Ann. Stat. §§ 191.300-.380 (1991) (genetics and metabolic disease programs); N.J. Stat. Ann. §§ 26:5B-1-4 (1991) (hereditary disorders); Tenn. Code Ann. §§ 68-5-501-505 (1991) (genetics program); Tex. Health & Safety Code Ann. §§ 134.001-.007 (1991) (Interagency Council for Genetic Services); Va. Code §§ 32.1–68 & -69 (1990) (genetics program); Wash. Rev. Code Ann. §§ 70.83B.010-.900 (1990) (prenatal diagnosis).

89. See Boodman (1992); Pub. L. No. 100–578, 102 Stat. 2903 (1988), codified at 42 U.S.C.A. § 263a (1991).

90. Cal. Health & Safety Code § 309.5 (1991) (genetic disease fund); Cal. Health & Safety Code §1367.7 (1991) (health care service plan cover-

age of prenatal diagnosis); Cal. Ins. Code § 10123.9 (1991) (group policy coverage of prenatal diagnosis); Cal. Ins. Code § 11512.18 (1991) (nonprofit hospital service plan coverage of prenatal diagnosis); 1991 Cal. Stat. 1014, to be codified at Cal. Health & Safety Code § 309; La. Rev. Stat. Ann. § 215.8 (1991) (insurance for cleft lip/palate, if provided, must include genetic counseling); 1991 Minn. Ch. Laws 33, § 36 (some insurance benefits to cover prenatal diagnosis), to be codified at Minn. Stat. Ann. ch. 62K; Minn. R. § 9505.0235 (1991) (Medicaid will pay for ultrasound and laboratory tests to detect fetal abnormalities); 1991 Mont. Laws 638 (insurers to pay fee to fund genetic services), codified at Mont. Code Ann. § 33-2-712 (1992); Wash. Rev. Code Ann. § 48.21.244 (1990) (group disability to pay for prenatal diagnosis); Wash. Rev. Code Ann. § 48.44.344 (1990) (group health care services contract to cover prenatal diagnosis); Wash. Rev. Code Ann. § 48.46.375 (1990) (HMOs to cover prenatal diagnosis).

91. Ohio Rev. Code Ann. § 3111.33 (1992).

BIBLIOGRAPHY

ANDREWS, L. B. (1987). *Medical genetics: A legal frontier.* Chicago: American Bar Foundation.

BOODMAN, S. G. (1992, September). Errors in genetic tests. *Washington Post* (p. Z11).

CLAYTON, E. W. (1992). Screening and treatment of newborns. *Houston Law Review, 29,* 85–148.

CONGREGATION for the Doctrine of Faith. (1987). Instruction on respect for human life in its origin and on the dignity of procreation: Replies to certain questions of the day. In R. R. Hull (Ed.), *Ethical issues in the new reproductive technologies* (pp. 21–39). Belmont, CA: Wadsworth.

CUNNINGHAM, G. C. (1990). Balancing the individual's rights to privacy against the need for information to protect and advance public health. In B. M. Knoppers & C. M. Laberge (Eds.), *Genetic screening: From newborns to DNA typing* (pp. 239–252). New York: Excerpta Medica.

HICKSON, G. B., Clayton, E. W., Githens, P. B., & Sloan, F. A. (1992). Factors that prompted families to file medical claims following prenatal injuries. *Journal of the American Medical Association, 267,* 1359–1363.

HOOD, H. A., Kavass, I., & Galvin, C. O. (Eds.). (1991). *Abortion in the United States: A compilation of state legislation.* Buffalo: William S. Hein.

KARJALA, D. S. (1992). A legal research agenda for the human genome initiative. *Jurimetrics, 32,* 121–222.

LIPPMAN, A. (1991). Prenatal genetic testing and screening: Constructing needs and reinforcing inequities. *American Journal of Law and Medicine, 17,* 15–50.

REILLY, P. (1987). *Genetics, law, and social policy*. Cambridge, MA: Harvard University Press.

REILLY, P. (1991). *The surgical solution*. Baltimore: Johns Hopkins University Press.

ROTHMAN, B. K. (1986). *The tentative pregnancy*. New York: Penguin.

SLOAN, F. A., Githens, P. B., Clayton, E. W., Hickson, G. B., Gentile, D. A., & Partlett, D. F. (Eds.). (1993). *Suing for malpractice*. Chicago: University of Chicago Press.

WRIGHT, E. E. (1978). Father and mother know best: Defining the liability of physicians for inadequate genetic counseling. *Yale Law Journal, 87*, 1488–1515.

APPENDIX

TABLE 1 **Statutes and Regulations Addressing Genetic Services**

State	General Genetics Program	Part of New-born Screening?	Specific Disease	Prenatal Diagnosis	Medical Assistance	Private Insurance
AL (s)	Y v			Y v		
CA (s) *	Y f			Y	Y p	Y p
CO (s)	Y f	Y				
FL (s)		Y	Y e			
GA (s)	Y n					
HI (s)				Y		
IL (s) m						
IL (r)	Y mch			Y mch		
IO (s)(r) e	Y c					
KS (s) ch			Y c			
KY (s) m mt						
LA (s) e d			Y cl n			Y cl
LA (r)	Y					
ME (s)	Y n			Y		
MD (s) d	Y f		Y			
MD (r)	Y			Y ntd		
MA (s)	Y f					
MI (s) educ	Y n		Y			
MN (s) fp	Y e n				Y p	Y p
MN (r)						Y p
MO (s)	Y c		Y	Y nr	Y	
MT (s) d	Y v	Y				Y sur
NV (s)	Y c			Y		

(continued)

TABLE 1 (*continued*)

State	General Genetics Program	Part of New-born Screen-ing?	Specific Disease	Prenatal Diagnosis	Medical Assis-tance	Private Insur-ance
NJ (s) m d	Y ?					
NY (s) d	Y n					
NC (s)		Y				
NC (r)	Y					
ND (s) be						
OH (s)	Y ? n					
OH (r)	Y mch			Y mch		
OR (s)				Y v		
PA (s)			Y			
PR (s)		Y				
TN (s)	Y c			Y na		
TX (s)	Y n					
UT (s)	Y n			Y ns		
VA (s) m	Y c					
WA (s)	Y n				Y p	Y p
WA (r)				Y		
WI (r)	Y fp			Y fp		

LEGEND

be calling for bioethics commission
c confidentiality
ch parents to be told about possibility of testing children for
    sickle-cell trait upon their entry to school
cl required only for families of patients with cleft lip &/or palate
d antidiscrimination law addressing genetics
e eugenic language
educ provides for education in schools
f far reaching statement of protection of patients
fp family planning services include genetic counseling
m information regarding genetics given to applicants for marriage licenses

mch maternal child health program

mt physicians to test marriage applicants for sickle-cell disease or trait

n no statement regarding protection of patients

na cannot do prenatal diagnosis of diseases for which there is no treatment

nr cannot refer for abortion unless continuing pregnancy would threaten life of mother

ns "program of prenatal diagnosis for the purpose of detecting the possible or handicaps of an unborn child will not be used for screening, but rather will be utilized only when there are medical or genetic indications which warrant diagnosis"

ntd neural tube defects/MSAFP

p prenatal diagnosis

r regulation

s statute

sur surcharge placed on insurers to pay for state genetics program

v voluntary

* comprehensive program including education in schools

? discusses hereditary diseases but does not really address screening and counseling

STATUTES AND REGULATIONS REFERRED TO BY STATE

Alabama (statute)
Ala. Code §§ 22–10A-1-3 (1991) (genetics program).

California (statute)
Cal. Educ. Code §§ 51780–51782 (1991) (education in schools).
Cal. Health & Safety Code §§ 150–156.3 (1991) (Hereditary Diseases Act and prenatal diagnosis).
Cal. Health & Safety Code § 309.5 (1991) (genetic disease fund).
Cal. Health & Safety Code §1367.7 (1991) (health care service plan coverage of prenatal diagnosis).
Cal. Ins. Code § 10123.9 (1991) (group policy coverage of prenatal diagnosis).
Cal. Ins. Code § 11512.18 (1991) (nonprofit hospital service plan coverage of prenatal diagnosis).
1991 Cal. Stat. 1014, to be codified at Cal. Health & Safety Code § 309.
1992 Cal. Stat. 794, to be codified at Cal. Health & Safety Code § 309.

Colorado (statute)
Colo. Rev. Stat. §§ 25-4-1001-1006 (1991) (Newborn Screening and Genetic Counseling and Education Act).

Florida (statute)
Fla. Stat. Ann. § 393.064 (1991) (developmental disabilities of genetic origin).

Georgia (statute)
Ga. Code Ann. § 31-12-5 (1991) (medical genetics services).

Hawaii (statute)
Hawaii Rev. Stat. § 321–331 (1990) (prenatal diagnosis).

Illinois (statute)
20 Ill. Comp. Stat. Ann. § 2310/55.55 (1993) (brochure for applicants for
marriage license).

Illinois (regulation)
77 Ill. Admin. Code § 630.30 (1985) (MCH project to cover genetic
screening and prenatal diagnosis).

Iowa (statute and regulation)
Iowa Code Ann. §§ 136A.1–7 (1991) (Birth Defects Institute).
1990 Iowa Senate Joint Res. 2003 (genetic factors among those contributions
to developmental disability that can be "prevented or minimized").
Iowa Admin. Code §§ 136A.1-.7 (1983) (genetics program).

Kansas (statute)
Kan. Stat. Ann. §§ 65–1,105b–1,106 (1990) (sickle-cell testing including
advising parents of new school entrants of possibility of testing).

Kentucky (statute)
Ky. Rev. Stat. Ann. §§ 402.310-.990 (1991) (requiring that physicians test
applicants for marriage license for sickle-cell disease/trait).

Louisiana (statute)
La. Rev. Stat. Ann. § 23:1002 (1991) (anti-discrimination; sickle-cell trait).
La. Rev. Stat. Ann. § 28:381(16) (1991) (genetic counseling for families of
mentally retarded or developmentally disabled).
La. Rev. Stat. Ann. § 22:215.8 (1991) (insurance for cleft lip/palate, if
provided, must include genetic counseling).

Louisiana (regulation)
La. Admin. Code §§ 6501–3, 6901–3 (1987) (genetics program and advisory
committee).

Maine (statute)
Me. Rev. Stat. Ann. tit. 22, § 1533 (1989) (genetics program).

Maryland (statute)
Md. Pub. Health Code Ann. §18–503 (1991) (sickle-cell anemia).
Md. Ann. Code art 48A, §223 (1991) (anti-discrimination).
Md. Pub. Health Code Ann. §§ 13-101-111 (1991) (Hereditary and
Congenital Disorders Program).

Maryland (regulation)
Md. Admin. Code tit. 10, §§ 39.02.01-.10, 39.03.01-.06, 52.01.01-.06
(genetics programs and MSAFP).

Massachusetts (statute)
Mass. Gen. Laws Ann. ch. 76, § 15B (1991) (genetic screening).

Michigan (statute)
Mich. Comp. Laws Ann. §§ 333.5401-.5439 (1991) (chronic disease
program, which includes genetics).
Mich. Comp. Laws Ann. § 380.1507 (1991) (some genetic information may
be included within school sex education programs).

Minnesota (statute)
Minn. Stat. Ann. § 144.91 (1991) (genetics program).

Minn. Stat. Ann. § 145.925 (1991) (genetic counseling as part of family planning).
1991 Minn. Ch. Laws 33, § 36 (some insurance benefits to cover prenatal diagnosis), to be codified at Minn. Stat. Ann. ch. 62K.

Minnesota (regulation)
Minn. R. § 9505.0235 (1991) (Medicaid will pay for ultrasound and laboratory tests to detect fetal abnormalities).

Missouri (statute)
Mo. Ann. Stat. §§ 191.300–.380 (1991) (genetics and metabolic disease programs).

Montana (statute)
Mont. Code Ann. § 33-18-206 (1991), as amended by, 1991 Mont. Laws 318 (anti-discrimination).
Mont. Code Ann. § 50-19-211 (1991) (voluntary genetics program).
1991 Mont. Laws 638 (insurers to pay fee to fund genetic services), codified at Mont. Code Ann. § 33-2-712 (1992).

Nevada (statute)
1991 Nev. Stat. 622 (genetics program, including prenatal diagnosis), codified at Nev. Rev. Stat. Ann. §§ 396.521–.527 (1991).

New Jersey (statute)
N.J. Stat. Ann. §§ 26:5B-1-4 (1991) (hereditary disorders).
N.J. Stat. Ann. § 37:1–27 (1991) (brochures to applicants for marriage licenses).

New York (statute)
N.Y. Pub. Health Law §§ 2730–2733 (1991) (Birth Defects Institute).
N.Y. Civ. Rights Law §§ 48–48b (1991) (anti-discrimination).

North Carolina (statute)
N.C. Gen. Stat. § 95–28.1 (1991) (anti-discrimination; sickle-cell trait or hemoglobin C trait).

North Carolina (regulation)
N.C. Admin. Code tit. 15A, §§ 21H.0301–.0313 (1991) (genetics program).

North Dakota (statute)
1989 N.D. Senate Concurrent Resolution 4055 (calling for bioethics study).

Ohio (statute)
Ohio Rev. Code Ann. § 3701.502 (1989) (genetics program).

Ohio (regulation)
Ohio Admin. Code §§ 5101:3-4-07&08 (1989) (genetics within family planning and obstetrical services).

Oregon (statute)
Or. Rev. Stat. §§ 352.055–.058 (1991) (genetics program and prenatal diagnosis).

Pennsylvania (statute)
1991 Pa. Law 40-A & 1992 Pa. Law 34A (establishing program for Tay-Sachs at Jefferson Medical College).

Puerto Rico (statute)
P.R. Laws Ann. 24, § 3156 (1990) (genetic counseling associated with
newborn screening).

Tennessee (statute)
Tenn. Code Ann. §§ 68-5-501-505 (1991) (genetics program).

Texas (statute)
Tex. Health & Safety Code Ann. §§ 134.001-.007 (1991) (Interagency
Council for Genetic Services).

Utah (statute)
Utah Code Ann. § 26-5-2 (1990) (genetics program as part of effort to
prevent chronic disease).
Utah Code Ann. § 26-10-1 (1990) (suggesting that some prenatal diagnosis
may be provided under maternal/child health).

Virginia (statute)
Va. Code § 20–14.2 (1990) (information of applicants for marriage licenses).
Va. Code §§ 32.1–68&69 (1990) (genetics program).

Washington (statute)
Wash. Rev. Code Ann. § 48.21.244 (1990) (group disability to pay for
prenatal diagnosis).
Wash. Rev. Code Ann. § 48.44.344 (1990) (group health care services
contract to cover prenatal diagnosis).
Wash. Rev. Code Ann. § 48.46.375 (1990) (HMOs to cover prenatal
diagnosis).
Wash. Rev. Code Ann. § 70-54-220 (1993) (requiring practitioners to inform
patients about prenatal tests).

Washington (regulation)
Wash. Admin. Code R. §§ 246-680-001-020 (1990) (prenatal diagnosis).

Wisconsin (regulation)
Wis. Admin. Code § HSS 107.21 (1986) (family planning includes range of
services including prenatal diagnosis).

TABLE 2 Wrongful Birth and Wrongful Life Damages

State (Level of Authority) Citation	Wrongful Birth				Wrong-ful Life
	Full Eco-nomic Damages	Extraor-dinary Damages	Emo-tional Damages	Minus Benefits	
AL (S) *Elliot v. Brown*, 361 So.2d 546 (1978)					N
AL (F) *Robak v. U.S.*, 658 F.2d 471 (7th Cir.) (1981)	Y				
AZ (S) *Walker v. Mart*, 790 P.2d 735 (1990)		D ?			N
CA (S) *Turpin v. Sortini*, 643 P.2d 954 (1982)					Y *
CA (I) *Turpin v. Sortini*, 643 P.2d 954 (1982)		P	N		
CA (I) *Andalon v. Super Ct.*, 208 Cal. Rptr. 899 (1984)					N #
CA Cal. Health & Safety Code § 43.6 (1991)					N @
CO (S) *Lininger v. Eisenbaum*, 764 P.2d 1202 (1988)		Y		A	N
CO Colo. Rev. Stat. § 13-64-502 (1991)		N			N

(continued)

TABLE 2 *(continued)*

State (Level of Authority) Citation	Wrongful Birth				Wrong-ful Life
	Full Eco-nomic Damages	Extraor-dinary Damages	Emo-tional Damages	Minus Benefits	
CT (S) *Ochs v. Borelli,* 445 A.2d 883 (1982)		Y	Y		
CT (I) *Donnelly v. Candlewood Obstet-Gynecol. Assoc.,* No. 30 20 96, 1992 Conn. Super. LEXIS 1682 (1992)					N
DC (I) *Haymon v. Wilkerson,* 535 A.2d 880 (1987)	NA	Y			NA
DE (S) *Garrison v. Medical Center of Del.,* 581 A.2d 288 (1990)		Y	N		N
FL (S) *Fassoulas v. Ramey,* 450 So.2d 984 (1984)	N	Y			
FL (S) *Kush v. Lloyd,* 616 So. 2d 415 (1992)		Y *	Y		

(continued)

TABLE 2 *(continued)*

State (Level of Authority) Citation	Wrongful Birth				Wrong-ful Life
	Full Eco-nomic Damages	Extraor-dinary Damages	Emo-tional Damages	Minus Benefits	
FL (I) *Moores v. Lucas,* 405 So.2d 1022 (1981)		Y		N	N
GA (S) *Atlanta Obstet.* *Gynecol. Group* *v. Abelson,* 398 S.E.2d 557 (1990)		N			NA
ID (S) *Blake v. Cruz,* 698 P.2d 315 (1984)		Y	Y	Y	N
ID Idaho Code § 5–334 (1991)		N ~			N ~
IL (S) *Sieminiec v.* *Lutheran Gen.* *Hosp.,* 512 N.E.2d 691 (1987)		Y	N		N
IL (S) *Goldberg v.* *Ruskin,* 499 N.E.2d 406 (1986)					N
IN (S) *Cowe v. Forum* *Grp.,* 575 N.E.2d 630 (1991)					N
IN Ind. Code Ann. § 34-1-1-11 (1991)					N ~

(continued)

TABLE 2 (*continued*)

State (Level of Authority) Citation	Wrongful Birth				Wrong-ful Life
	Full Eco-nomic Damages	Extraor-dinary Damages	Emo-tional Damages	Minus Benefits	

KS (S)
Arche v. U.S.,
  798 P.2d 477
  (1990)
		Y	N	N	

KS (S)
Bruggeman v.
  Schimke, 718
  P.2d 635
  (1986)
					N

LA (S)
Pitre v. Opelousas
  Gen. Hosp.,
  530 So.2d 1151
  (1988)
		N ¶			Y D

LA (I)
Pines v. Moreno,
  569 So.2d 203
  (La. App.
  1990)
		Y	Y		

ME
Me. Rev. Stat.
  Ann. tit. 24,
  § 2931 (1989)
		Y			Y

MA (S)
Viccaro v.
  Milunsky, 551
  N.E.2d 8
  (1990)
		Y	Y	Y	N

MI (I)
Proffit v. Bartolo,
  412 N.W.2d
  232 (1987)
		Y	Y		N

MI (I)
Strohmaier v.
  Assoc. Obstet.
  Gynecol., 332
  N.W.2d 432
  (1982)
					N

(*continued*)

TABLE 2 *(continued)*

State (Level of Authority) Citation	Wrongful Birth				Wrongful Life
	Full Economic Damages	Extraordinary Damages	Emotional Damages	Minus Benefits	
MI (I) *Dorlin v. Providence Hosp.*, 325 N.W.2d 600 (1982)					N
MI (I) *Eisbrenner v. Stanley*, 308 N.W.2d 209 (1981)		Y	Y		N
MN Minn. Stat. Ann. § 145.424 (1991)		N ~			N ~
MO (S) *Shelton v. St. Anthony's Med. Ctr.*, 781 S.W.2d 48 (1989)		N	Y^		
MO (S) *Wilson v. Kuenzi*, 751 S.W.2d 741 (1988)		N			N
MO Mo. Ann. Stat. § 188.130 (1991)		N ~			N ~
NH (S) *Smith v. Cote*, 513 A.2d 341 (1986)		Y			N
NJ (S) *Procanik v. Cillo*, 478 A.2d 755 (1984)					Y *

(continued)

TABLE 2   (*continued*)

State (Level of Authority) Citation	Wrongful Birth				Wrong-ful Life
	Full Eco-nomic Damages	Extraor-dinary Damages	Emo-tional Damages	Minus Benefits	
NJ (S) *Schroeder v.* *Perkel*, 432 A.2d 834 (1981)		Y			
NJ (S) *Berman v. Allan*, 404 A.2d 8 (1979)	N		Y		N r
NJ (S) *Hummel v. Reiss*, 608 A.2d 1341 (1992)					N +
NY (S) *Bani-Esraili v.* *Lerman*, 505 N.E.2d 947 (1987)		N post-21			
NY (S) *Alquijay v.* *St. Luke's-* *Roosevelt Hosp.* *Ctr.*, 473 N.E.2d 244 (1984)					N
NY (S) *Becker v.* *Schwartz*, 386 N.E.2d 807 (1978)		Y	N		N
NY (S) *Howard v.* *Lecher*, 366 N.E.2d 64 (1977)			N		

(*continued*)

TABLE 2 *(continued)*

State (Level of Authority) Citation	Wrongful Birth				Wrong-ful Life
	Full Eco-nomic Damages	Extraor-dinary Damages	Emo-tional Damages	Minus Benefits	
NC (S) *Azzolino v. Dingfelder*, 337 S.E.2d 528 (1985), cert. denied, 479 U.S. 835 (1986)		N			N
NC (F) *Gallagher v. Duke Univ.*, 852 F.2d 773 (4th Cir.) (1988)	Y	Y =	Y	N	
OK (S) *Spencer v. Seikel*, 742 P.2d 1126 (1987)		N			
PA (S) *Ellis v. Sherman*, 515 A.2d 1327 (1986)		D Y	D Y		N
PA (S) *Speck v. Finegold*, 439 A.2d 110 (1981)	Y		Y		N
PA (I) *Stribling v. deQuevedo*, 432 A.2d 239 (Pa. Super.) (1980)		Y	N r		N
PA Pa. Stat. Ann. tit. 42, § 8305 (1991)		N ~			N

(continued)

TABLE 2 *(continued)*

| State (Level of Authority) Citation | Wrongful Birth | | | | Wrongful Life |
	Full Economic Damages	Extraordinary Damages	Emotional Damages	Minus Benefits	
SC (F) (4 opinions) *Phillips v. U.S.*, 508 F. Supp. 537 (1980); *Phillips v. U.S.*, 508 F. Supp. 544 (1981); *Phillips v. U.S.*, 566 F. Supp. 1 (1981); *Phillips v. U.S.*, 575 F. Supp. 1309 (1983)	N	Y life expect	Y	Y	N
SD S. Dak. Codified Laws Ann. §§ 21-55-1 & -2 (1991)		N ~			N
TN (S) *Owens v. Foote*, 773 S.W.2d 911 (1989)		D Y			
TX (S) *Nelson v. Krusen*, 678 S.W.2d 918 (1984)					N
TX (S) *Jacobs v. Theimer*, 519 S.W.2d 846 (1975)		Y	D N		
UT Utah Code Ann. § 78-11-24 (1990)		N ~			N ~
VA (S) *Naccash v. Burger*, 290 S.E.2d 825 (1982)		Y	Y		

(continued)

TABLE 2 *(continued)*

State (Level of Authority) Citation	Wrongful Birth				Wrongful Life
	Full Economic Damages	Extraordinary Damages	Emotional Damages	Minus Benefits	
WA (S) *Harbeson v. Parke-Davis,* 656 P.2d 483 (1983); *Harbeson v. Parke-Davis,* 746 F.2d 517 (9th Cir.) (1984)		Y			Y *
WV (S) *James G. v. Caserta,* 332 S.E.2d 872 (1985)		Y			N
WI (S) *Dumer v. St. Michaels Hosp.,* 233 N.W. 2d 372 (1975)		Y			N

LEGEND

S state supreme court
I state appellate court
F federal court
Y yes
N no
D dicta
NA not appealed
P pending, awaiting trial below
r reversed by later opinion
* extraordinary expenses after majority
# no lost earning capacity
@ children barred from bringing claims only against parents
~ abortion only
¶ occurrence of genetic defect not foreseeable
^ can recover only for the emotional injury of not being warned that fetus had congenital defects
+ negligence occurred before *Roe v. Wade*
= medical expenses recoverable only until parents' death

TABLE 3 **Statutes that Address Abortion of Fetuses with Defects**

BEFORE VIABILITY

State	Statutory Language
Del. Code Ann. tit. 24, § 1790 (1991)	permissible reasons for abortion include "substantial risk of the birth of the child with grave and permanent physical deformity or mental retardation"
Idaho Code § 18–608 (1991)	factors physician is to consider in deciding whether to provide first or second trimester abortion include "that the child would be born with some physical or mental defect"
Kan. Stat. Ann. § 21–3407 (1991)	physician justified in performing abortion "if there is substantial risk that . . . the child would be born with physical or mental defect"
Md. Pub. Health Code Ann. § 20–208 (1991)	can perform abortion if "[t]here is substantial risk of the birth of the child with grave and permanent physical deformity or mental retardation"
N.H. Rev. Stat. Ann. § 585.13 (1991)	abortion of fetus after quickening is permissible if "malformation" in fetus would threaten the life of the woman
Pa. Cons. Stat. Ann. tit. 18, § 3204 (1991)	forbidding abortion "which is sought solely because of the sex of the unborn child"
Tex. Rev. Civ. Stat. Ann. art 44956 (1991)	physician can perform abortion if "the fetus has a severe and irreversible abnormality, as identified through reliable diagnostic procedures"
1991 Utah Laws ch. 2, codified at Utah Code Ann. §§ 76-7-301-317.1 (1992)	can perform abortion "if the unborn child would be born with grave defects"

THIRD TRIMESTER ABORTIONS

State	Statutory Language
Idaho Code § 18–608 (1991)	if abortion not performed, "pregnancy would terminate in birth or delivery of a fetus unable to survive"
Kan. Stat. Ann. § 21–3407 (1991)	can perform abortion if "there is substantial risk . . . that the child would be born with physical or mental defect" [no mention of viability]
Md. Pub. Health Code Ann. § 20–208 (1991)	can perform abortion if "[t]here is substantial risk of the birth of the child with grave and permanent physical deformity or mental retardation" until 26 weeks' gestation
N.H. Rev. Stat. Ann. § 585.13 (1991)	can perform abortion after quickening if fetal malformation would threaten life of woman
Tex. Rev. Civ. Stat. Ann. art 44956 (1991)	can perform abortion if the fetus "has a severe and irreversible abnormality, as identified through reliable diagnostic procedures"
1991 Utah Laws ch. 2, codified at Utah Code Ann. §§ 76-7-301-317.1 (1992)	can perform abortion "if the unborn child would be born with grave defects"

TABLE 4 **Statutes That Address Funding of Abortions of Fetuses with Defects**

State	Statutory Language
Colo. Rev. Stat. §§ 26-4-105.5 & 26-15-104.5 (1991)	"presence of a lethal medical condition in the unborn child . . . which would result in the impending death of the unborn child during the term of pregnancy or at birth"
1991 Iowa Acts 267, §§ 103,b & 210, o(2)	"fetus is physically deformed, mentally deficient, or afflicted with a congenital illness"
1992 Md. Laws 64, § 1, 32.17.01.02	"genetic defect or serious deformity or abnormality"
1992 Tenn. Pub. Act. 1018, § 10, Item 4(3)	fetus is "medically determined to have severe physical deformities or abnormalities or severe mental retardation"
Va. Code § 32.1–92.1 (1991)	"any case in which a physician who is trained and qualified to perform such tests certifies in writing, after appropriate tests have been performed, that he believes the fetus will be born with a gross and totally incapacitating physical deformity or with a gross and totally incapacitating mental deficiency"

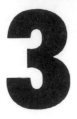

Psychological and Sociocultural Issues

The six chapters in this part delineate a variety of perspectives on the psychological and sociocultural issues raised by reproductive genetic testing. Elena Gates poses a series of questions on the benefits and burdens of prenatal testing on women, including its impact on anxiety, sense of control, and relationships with family. Are reproductive genetic tests carried out for the benefit of the woman, the fetus, or society? Do the availability and application of the tests enhance or diminish a woman's autonomy? Does testing increase rather than decrease the burdens of pregnancy? Does testing afford the promised reassurance or does it provide too much or too little reassuring information?

Sociocultural differences and similarities among consumers in relation to their decisions about reproductive genetic testing are examined in the next three chapters. The first of those chapters, by Nancy Press and Carole Browner, identifies factors that influence a woman's decision to accept or reject prenatal testing. Their findings suggest that the way in which women were informed and the kind of information they were given had a greater impact on their decision than did their ethnic or social-class background. They argue that because reproductive genetic testing is becoming a routine part of prenatal care, and because of implicit beliefs concerning the value of scientific knowledge, individuals in society are enabled, regardless of ethnic or social class, to remain silent about issues on which there is no societal consensus, such as abortion or genetic manipulation.

In contrast, Rayna Rapp describes her study of the social impact and cultural meaning of prenatal testing. Based on her anthropological study, she finds important ethnocultural and socioeconomic differences between providers and consumers. She concludes that providers must be sensitive to such diversity when delivering prenatal testing services.

Laurie Nsiah-Jefferson highlights the limited access to reproductive genetic testing faced by many low-income women, women of color, and geographically isolated women. She discusses barriers, not only to the specialized services, but to basic prenatal care. She further examines the difficulties created by lack of cultural sensitivity, perceived imbalance of power, and mistrust, which influence the provision (or lack) of genetic services.

The final two chapters refocus attention on the overall impact of reproductive genetic testing on women. Barbara Katz Rothman examines the ways in which prenatal diagnosis changes how a woman experiences pregnancy. In particular, she concludes that the pregnancy in its first half is overshadowed by the concern for what may happen in the second half. As a consequence, she argues that this "tentative pregnancy" is redefining the future of motherhood with increasing frequency.

Rita Beck Black then considers the experiences of women undergoing reproductive genetic testing, with special attention focused on the impact of pregnancy loss after testing. She discusses the way in which undergoing prenatal genetic testing can be a major psychological and social event for women, this being even more the case if the testing reveals a possible problem. She calls for further research in this area to provide a more in-depth understanding of the meaning of these experiences for women and their families.

9 Prenatal Genetic Testing:

Does It Benefit Pregnant Women?

ELENA A. GATES

Prenatal diagnosis of chromosomal abnormalities, neural tube defects, and specific genetic disorders is becoming increasingly available to pregnant women in this country. As the Human Genome Project yields more information about the genes responsible for illnesses, medical conditions that develop later in life, and basic human differences, and as medical science develops safer and simpler techniques for obtaining genetic material, the spectrum of conditions for which testing will be available will expand dramatically. Decisions about the appropriate use of these new tests and technologies will be challenging. This will especially be true when decisions about genetic testing intertwine with decisions made by women about reproduction, as occurs in the use of prenatal genetic testing.

In the general practice of medicine, it is important to consider not only therapeutic results, but also the nonclinical implications of what is done to or for patients. This is particularly imperative when one considers prenatal genetic screening and testing and its application to broad populations of women. A few basic questions need to be asked: Do we know whether prenatal genetic testing is a good thing for women, children, or society? Does prenatal genetic testing go beyond merely providing more information about a woman's pregnancy to actually improving her health? The term health is used broadly in this context, as described by *Dorland's Illustrated Medical Dictionary* (1988) as a "state of optimal physical, mental, and social well-being, not merely as the absence of disease and infirmity."

While it is clear that prenatal genetic testing is very useful for identifying a particular chromosomal or genetic abnormality in a fetus, and that it can offer meaningful choices to families at risk for specific genetic disorders, less evidence exists to indicate whether the widespread application of testing to pregnant women will succeed in achieving the broader goal of improving the health and well-being of obstetric patients. Indeed, several goals can be postulated for a broadly applied program of prenatal genetic testing.

Is Prenatal Diagnosis Intended to Benefit Society?

The notion that individual women should be offered or encouraged to undergo prenatal genetic testing in order to spare society the expense of coping with diseased or disabled offspring has been put forward (Shaw, 1984). Viewed in terms of medical economics, the burden of genetic diseases on society is significant. "Genetic disorders account for about 20 percent of pediatric hospital admissions and for an even higher percentage of long term admissions" (Simpson, 1986). Widespread application of prenatal genetic testing, if accompanied by treatment or by termination of pregnancy, would decrease the social burden of genetic disease, at least in economic terms. Currently, however, most diagnosable conditions are not treatable prenatally. Furthermore, access to abortion, even for diagnosed genetic conditions, may be limited, either legally, economically, or by inadequate availability of abortion services in certain areas of the country.

Even if prenatal diagnostic testing could decrease the social burden of genetic disease by preventing the birth of affected individuals, it is not clear that our society is ready to promote prenatal genetic testing in conjunction with abortion primarily for this end. In statistical terms, the selective abortion of fetuses affected with genetically determined conditions would in fact increase the prevalence of abnormal genes in the population if fetuses found to be carriers of recessive conditions were spared

(Boss, 1990). Furthermore, it is unlikely that decreasing the rate of genetic disease would address the ills of society as effectively as other sorts of social measures such as improved access to health care or education. Even more important, the limitations to individual reproductive freedom required by a program of mandatory screening and termination of pregnancy would be intolerable.

Does Prenatal Genetic Testing Provide a Benefit to the Child?

Benefit to the expected child can be achieved in some situations. If the diagnosed condition is one treatable before birth, the future child should benefit. For example, there has been some success in treating alpha thalassemia and combined immunodeficiency syndromes by fetal bone marrow transplantation. If the condition diagnosed will impact obstetric or prenatal management, the future child may benefit. For example, if hemophilia is diagnosed in a fetus, scalp sampling and the use of a vacuum extractor to assist in delivery can be avoided for fear of injuring the child. However, when no treatment exists and pregnancy termination is the only alternative to doing nothing, there may be no benefit to the child. Whether being spared a life with disease, pain, or disability is a benefit to the child is a difficult ethical question on which a spectrum of articulate opinions exists (Botkin, 1988; Elias & Annas, 1987; Liu, 1987).

Is Prenatal Genetic Testing Intended to Benefit Women?

When one studies the impact of a medical intervention on the health or the quality of life of patients, the approach is typically to assess the relative burdens and benefits of the intervention in question. Another consideration is whether and in what ways prenatal genetic testing is intended to benefit the parents (or more specifically, the mother) of the future child. Prenatal diagnosis may in some ways enhance the quality of life for women, both during and after pregnancy. It may be useful in allowing a woman to have the choice of whether to bear a child with a genetic or other congenital disorder. Further, it may provide the pregnant woman with needed information about the medical condition of her fetus. However, there may also be risks involved such as an increased anxiety, leading to a reduction in her quality of life. The practice of prenatal diagnosis can be expected to impact women in a number of ways, and it is not absolutely apparent that all of these impacts are positive. In fact, what is construed as a benefit for one woman may on the contrary be burdensome for another. Experiences will vary among women depending upon their individual backgrounds, experiences, and values.

Although the published data on the scientific aspects of prenatal diagnosis are extensive, significantly less data are available to demonstrate whether prenatal testing is truly beneficial or harmful to women's health in a broad sense. The majority of the data currently available relate to the prenatal diagnosis of chromosomal abnormalities and neural tube defects. Much less work has been done thus far on the impact of prenatal testing for specific genetic disorders. Even so, some interesting trends are apparent, and some preliminary questions about the less tangible effects of widespread prenatal genetic testing can be posed.

Is Prenatal Genetic Testing Reassuring?

One possible benefit of prenatal genetic testing might be to reassure a pregnant woman that the child she expects will be normal. This benefit has been widely promoted by advocates of testing. Consider, however, what role the availability of testing itself may have had in creating or sustaining the need for testing and reassurance. Are healthy women, entering the natural stage of pregnancy, being labeled "at risk" as a result of the development of tests for rare but potentially disabling genetic disorders?

There is evidence that prenatal testing, at least chromosomal and alpha-fetoprotein (AFP) testing, is reassuring to most women (Finley, Varner, Vinson, & Finley, 1977; Dixson et al., 1981; Robinson et al., 1988). There are, however, also indications that testing can raise anxiety prior to the procedure, reducing it if the results are normal (Beeson & Golbus, 1979).

The aspect of testing found to be most distressing has been the need to wait for results (Finley et al., 1977; Dixson et al., 1981; Evers-Kiebooms, Swerts, & Van den Berghe, 1988). One study found that a group of women who received an abnormally low result on AFP screening were noted to be significantly more worried about their baby's health three weeks after testing (after normal follow-up results were available) than were women who received normal results initially. Those differences were not appreciable at later points in the pregnancy (Marteau et al., 1992). According to other studies, it is not clear whether women who have undergone prenatal testing are left with less anxiety than those untested, once normal results are received (Tabor & Jonsson, 1987; Phipps & Zinn, 1986).

Prenatal diagnosis use may, in the end, raise more concerns about the pregnancy than it can answer. In deciding whether to have testing done, a woman must face the possibility of an untoward outcome when, in fact, her chances of having a normal infant are very high. Dixson followed women who received genetic counseling and then either underwent amniocentesis or declined. The rate of continuing concern about possible congenital abnormalities was just over 20% in both the group who received normal amniocentesis results and the group who declined testing (1981). Evers-Kiebooms (1988) found that one third of women tested felt reassured only after their child had been born. Although some women will experience residual anxiety, others will show more positive responses than had they not received reassurance from the test results.

The issue of reassurance can be examined in the converse. Can the information that is obtained through prenatal diagnosis be falsely reassuring? Even if the specific diagnosis being sought, such as for muscular dystrophy, is ruled out, there remains a two to three percent chance that the child will be born with some other kind of congenital disorder or genetic disease. Will women who undergo prenatal genetic testing be more or less prepared for other congenital problems that may arise? With the availability of testing, are women more inclined to focus on what may go wrong in a pregnancy rather than on the fact that things usually go right? While prenatal genetic testing may be valuable and reassuring for that group of women in whom significant risk for a specific abnormality exists, more data is needed before concluding that testing is on the whole reassuring to women.

Does Prenatal Genetic Testing Enhance the Autonomy of Pregnant Women?

Eric Cassell (1977), a physician and medical ethicist, has stated that "the primary function of medicine is to preserve, to repair, and to restore the patient's autonomy." While prenatal genetic testing does provide options to women at risk for bearing children with genetic diseases, it is not clear from existing data about reproductive choice that patient autonomy is actually enhanced through testing.

There is evidence that testing is, for some women, associated with a sense that control over important reproductive decisions is, to a degree, being usurped by family, by society, and by the medical profession. Berit Sjogren (1988) used a combination of questionnaires and interviews to assess whether women undergoing amniocentesis or chorionic villi sampling (CVS) made autonomous decisions regarding their testing. Most of the women surveyed (75%) found it difficult to refrain from prenatal diagnosis when it was offered. Seventy-eight percent felt it would be more difficult to give birth to a disabled child if they had not accepted prenatal diagnosis. Many stated that while they felt "free from external pressure," they still felt an "obligation" to have testing performed. Among women of a certain age, willingness to undergo prenatal diagnosis seems to be construed as a sign of responsible parenting. Is a woman acting irresponsibly in the eyes of others if prenatal diagnosis is foregone? Might a woman sense less sympathy and support if testing is foregone or if a pregnancy is continued in the face of adverse results? If perceptions such as these are common among pregnant women, the availability of prenatal diagnosis may indeed limit autonomy rather than enhance it.

To the extent that prenatal genetic testing actually provides women with the choice of whether to bear children with specific abnormalities, it does enhance their autonomy. If a specific disorder is diagnosable, it can be ruled out in a fetus. However, the woman may then be left with unrealistic ideas as to the chance of a different sort of disorder existing in her child. Will her ability to make responsible choices be limited by unrealistic expectations? How well will she be able to adjust if her child is affected with a disorder for which testing was not done? These questions remain unanswered.

The availability of prenatal genetic testing has brought the interests and influence of family, friends, and society into an individual woman's pregnancy to an increasing degree. Wertz (1992) found, in asking couples who had children affected with cystic fibrosis (CF) about prenatal testing for that condition, that "respondents' perceptions of their siblings' approval of abortion for CF was the best predictor of use of prenatal diagnosis." The opinions of the spouse and members of the extended family were also influential. Prenatal genetic testing appears to have opened the door to third-party involvement in the most private of decisions being made by women during pregnancy. Whether a woman chooses one form of childbirth preparation over another is an important decision but not fundamentally a moral one. Whether she has prenatal genetic testing and, further, what she decides to do with the information she receives may be one of the most serious moral decisions she will ever make. Involvement by parties such as employers and insurance companies in an individual woman's decisions about prenatal genetic testing will restrict reproductive choice in an unprecedented way (Gates, 1990).

In one illustrative case, a pregnant woman whose living child was affected with cystic fibrosis sought prenatal testing for the disease. When testing revealed that the expected child would also be affected with CF, the woman and her husband faced an agonizing decision. They ultimately decided not to abort the fetus. Their insurance company, an HMO, had agreed to extend special coverage for this woman's prenatal testing. It decided, however, that it would not provide medical coverage for an affected child, a child who would be born with a "preexisting condition" on account of the prenatal diagnostic procedure. As one journalist wrote, "The insurance company's message was clear: The parents could either abort the defective baby or struggle alone with the financial burden of a sick child" (Thompson, 1989). Although the HMO ultimately capitulated and agreed to cover the child's treatment, their initial policy serves as a sign of the new limits on maternal choice, which may evolve as the capacity for prenatal diagnosis expands. In the setting of widely available prenatal genetic testing, reproductive choices may become as much social choices as personal ones. It will be important to assess the impact of such testing on women's sense of their ability to retain control over the choices made about their pregnancies.

Is the Impact of Prenatal Genetic Testing Influenced by Issues Concerning Access to Family Planning Services?

At the same time that state legislatures around the country are planning and establishing programs to enable women through genetic screening and prenatal diagnosis to avoid conceiving or bearing affected children, a trend toward restricting a woman's right to decide to abort an affected fetus is evident. It seems likely, in view of recent Supreme Court decisions, that individual state legislatures will have increasing power to define the circumstances under which abortion will be legally available.[1] If access to abortion is significantly restricted, one really must ask just what kind of choices prenatal genetic testing offers. How much benefit is knowledge in the absence of meaningful options?

Although many are currently optimistic that abortion will remain a legal option in this country, women are still faced with significant limitations on the accessibility of abortion services both in financial terms and in terms of the number and geographical distribution of facilities offering abortion procedures. Women facing the termination of a desired pregnancy based on an abnormal result from prenatal testing may have even more difficulty because they must locate facilities that offer termination of second-trimester pregnancies.

Are the Choices Offered by Prenatal Genetic Testing Burdens in Themselves?

It is likely that the decisions required by the availability of prenatal genetic testing may be perceived as burdensome by some women. As Rayna Rapp (1987) has framed the question,

"Does amniocentesis offer women a 'window of control', or an anxiety-provoking responsibility?" Certainly, freedom and responsibility go hand in hand. Many women are able to make an informed decision to accept the burdens associated with testing in order to obtain the knowledge they seek. If testing is offered routinely and on a widespread basis, however, an informed and thoughtful decision may not be encouraged, and the burdens of testing may be both unexpected and troublesome.

If the test results indicate an abnormality, the woman must decide how to proceed—what to do with the information she has received. In Sjogren's study in Stockholm (1988), half the women surveyed stated that when they received their test result they had not yet reached a decision about what to do in the case of a fetal abnormality. Dixson (1981) found that one-third of the women surveyed remained uncertain at the time results were received. Adding to the complexity of the issue, at times the abnormality diagnosed prenatally, whether by chromosomal analysis, ultrasound, or specific genetic testing, is one for which the implications and prognosis are unclear. Thus, if a woman chooses to continue her pregnancy, anxiety about the outcome may be heightened; and if she elects termination of the pregnancy, she may wonder whether her decision was indeed the "right" one. In a group of patients surveyed by Drugan (1990), 93% of patients whose fetuses were diagnosed with a disorder bearing a severe prognosis elected to terminate their pregnancy. Twenty-seven percent of those with a questionable prognosis made this decision.

What Is the Impact of Prenatal Genetic Testing on a Woman's Relationships with Family and with Her Future Child?

The decisions a woman is required to make regarding prenatal genetic testing can be very stressful ones for her and for her partner. For many couples, this stress comes at a time when their relationship is already being redefined by the expectation of a child. The woman's partner may want prenatal diagnosis more than she does, and may be less anxious about it (Evans et al., 1988; Keenan, Basso, Goldkrand, & Butler, 1991), potentially leading the woman to experience a sense that "he'll blame

me if the child has a diagnosable abnormality that we don't find
out about," or "he'll blame me if we have an amniocentesis
complication." If the fetus is affected by a genetic disorder, the
woman and her partner may also feel different about the prospect of abortion. Those differences may impact a couple's relationship far into the future, regardless of the decision they ultimately make. The disagreement may furthermore affect their
relationship with the child, if the pregnancy is continued. The
integrity of these relationships is clearly important to women's
overall health. Little work has been done in terms of delineating
the effects of decisions about prenatal diagnosis on a woman's
family relationships. It will be important to clarify such ramifications before widespread testing is initiated.

Taken as a whole, investigation of amniocentesis's impact
suggests that anticipation of the procedure and its results may
lead to disruption of an otherwise normal adjustment to pregnancy. Studies have revealed that women undergoing amniocentesis may experience a "suspension of commitment to pregnancy" while awaiting test results (Beeson & Golbus, 1979;
Spencer & Cox, 1988). Beeson and Golbus (1979) observed that
this was reflected both in social spheres, such as in not telling
others about the pregnancy, and in personal domains, such as in
avoiding thinking about the pregnancy. Rothman (1986) noted
a greater frequency of women not feeling movement until after
the 18th week among those undergoing amniocentesis. In contrast, Dixson (1981) could demonstrate no significant differences between amniocentesis and nonamniocentesis groups in
the timing of selecting names or in willingness to talk about
the pregnancy. Furthermore, Phipps and Zinn (1986) found that
amniocentesis patients in a United States sample showed a
greater increase in fetal attachment over the course of pregnancy
than did nontested controls. Caccia (1991) demonstrated that
maternal-fetal attachment increased significantly for amniocentesis and CVS patients once normal results were received. No
nontested controls were included. It has also been noted that
attachment may be enhanced by viewing the fetus on ultrasound, a technology used in conjunction with amniocentesis
(Fletcher, 1983). If suspension of commitment does occur for
some women during the early months of pregnancy and if it

involves decreased compliance with suggested regimens such as good nutrition and abstaining from alcohol use, long-term adverse effects might result. Further investigation could clarify which women are at risk for this type of response to prenatal testing and could lead to meaningful interventions.

Jeffrey Botkin (1990) states that "a fundamental aspect of parenting is the recognition of the unique and independent nature of our children's personalities and lives. Try as we might, they rarely fit the molds that we design for them. A knowledge that our intrinsic personal characteristics were the intentional product of our parents' designs would have a profound influence on the parent-child relationship." Abby Lippman (1991) points out that "prenatal diagnosis does approach children as consumer objects subject to quality control." Those observations will be important to consider as the use of prenatal genetic testing expands. It will be important to clarify our understanding of women's expectations in relation to their children, as they depart from the illusion that they actually have some control over the "quality" of the infants they bear.

What Influence Does the Health Care Provider Have over the Effects of Prenatal Genetic Testing on Women?

The physician who counsels a woman about testing or about her response to abnormal results will have an important impact on her decision. Physicians may express, explicitly or implicitly, certain expectations about a woman's response to an adverse diagnosis. A woman, valuing her relationship with her physician and being in a relatively less powerful position in the physician–patient relationship, may hesitate to go against her physician's recommendations. If prenatal genetic testing becomes widespread, it will be essential that obstetricians become skilled in counseling women as they confront stressful decisions. A balance must be developed between supporting a woman through a difficult decision and limiting her ability to make her own choice. Holmes-Seidel (1987) reported an increased tendency for women to terminate a pregnancy affected by a sex chromosome abnormality when counseled by a general obstetrician rather than a geneticist. It is not clear how expert general obstetricians currently are at counseling women about genetic problems, nor is it clear that a balanced view about the disorders is presented by providers who have little or no personal experience with individuals who have disabilities.

When prenatal diagnostic testing is provided for a woman who is carrying a fetus at increased risk for a particular genetic condition, pretest and posttest genetic counseling are essential. The importance of the nonclinical implications of test results, and the acknowledgment that an individual woman's personal values are of primary importance are two considerations that underlie the concept of nondirective genetic counseling as practiced by most geneticists and genetics counselors. Currently, good pretest counseling consists of the provision of accurate information about the testing techniques involved and about the conditions being studied (Hsia & Hirschhorn, 1979). This information needs to be offered by an individual who has not only a solid knowledge of the science of genetics but also a familiarity with the particular condition being discussed. Once the information has been provided, the couple then goes on to make a decision about whether to have testing done and about which technique they would prefer. Such standards for genetic counseling have been developed with good reason: to ensure the benefits of genetic testing and, more important, to protect the individuals being tested from harm.

To date, a counselor has been able to focus on one or two conditions in counseling. A couple may, for example, want CVS to rule out chromosomal aneuploidy in addition, perhaps, to testing for a particular condition for which their fetus is at increased risk, such as muscular dystrophy. In the future, what will be offered may be a battery of tests for a spectrum of conditions of variable severity and for which an individual fetus or couple may not be at increased risk. The counseling challenge will be magnified. With broader application of prenatal genetic testing, the capacity of the current system for genetic counseling will be overwhelmed. A recent survey reveals that as many as 39% of the genetics counseling job openings in this country this year will probably not be filled because the number of individuals graduating from training programs is inadequate (Meyer, Edwards, Young, & Brooks, 1992). As a result, more and more of the burden of patient education and genetic counseling will fall to general obstetric providers.

It is worth considering how the genetic counseling model might be translated into a busy general obstetrics and gynecology practice where newly pregnant women and women planning a pregnancy are seen. The provider, whether obstetrician-gynecologist, midwife, or nurse-practitioner, is typically faced with a large volume of patients in order to satisfy patient demand and meet overhead expenses. Time constraints are a problem. Most important, the patients have many physical and psychological needs to be met. Providing information about tests for genetic conditions for which patients may not be at increased risk will probably not be a top priority in most situations, except perhaps when a woman comes specifically for fertility consultation, preconception counseling, or for an initial patient visit.

There is evidence that women's health care providers generally are not as skilled as trained genetic counselors, either in genetic knowledge or in the technique of counseling. For example, a survey of residents in obstetrics and gynecology in the Philadelphia area indicates that while most residents did have fairly good knowledge of teratology, those individuals scored, on average, between 54 and 65% correct on questions about clinical genetics and genetic testing (Kershner, Hammond, & Donnenfeld, 1992). If these results are representative, it is apparent that obstetrician-gynecologists will need to broaden their understanding of genetics before they will be able to inform patients adequately about the testing options and results available to them. One must also acknowledge that providers are under pressure to learn more about other important areas such as hormonal replacement in menopause, the evaluation and treatment of cervical intraepithelial lesions, and to improve their skill in the use of new technologies such as Norplant placement and endoscopic surgery. All of these areas are important to women's health, as much if not more so than is prenatal genetic testing.

Possible Approaches

In deciding which tests to start offering on a widespread basis and when, it will be important to keep in mind that testing should be performed with the intent of doing more than merely identifying randomly selected conditions in a limited number of women. Testing should be aimed at improving the health of women in the broadest sense. There is both a scientific and a moral obligation to demonstrate that prenatal genetic testing achieves this end effectively. Not only do studies on prenatal genetic diagnosis need to answer the scientific and practical questions (can the diagnosis be made accurately? can appropriate follow-up for results be provided?), they should also assess whether testing is beneficial to those who are meant to benefit, and whether testing results in significant harm to any parties.

Recent reports published about triple marker screening, for example, focus on the test's ability to identify fetuses with the targeted condition (Phillips et al., 1992; Haddow et al., 1992). As the use of this kind of screening is investigated further, and before such screening is offered on a widespread basis, attention needs to be devoted to assessing its impact on women in terms of their psychological adaptation to pregnancy, their sense of control over the outcome of their pregnancy, and their relationship with family. The impact of counseling on a woman's reactions to testing should also be studied further, including finding ways of enhancing a woman's sense of autonomy in making decisions about prenatal diagnosis, and the impact of prenatal "quality control" on a woman's relationship with her infant and child. Models like those used for quality of life assessment in clinical trials on disorders such as cancer and arthritis can be applied to trials of prenatal genetic diagnosis (Feeny & Torrance, 1989).

Providers of health care to women, whether physicians, midwives, or nurse-practitioners, will need to be educated more thoroughly about the principles of genetics, the nature of the conditions for which widespread testing is available, and the alternatives open to women who learn that their fetus is affected with a genetic condition. It is particularly important that those providers become skilled at counseling women in a manner which enhances their understanding of the tests being offered while enabling them to make thoughtful and uncoerced decisions about the use of this new technology.

Conclusion

In summary, two points should be recognized. First, there is not yet clear evidence of the impact that prenatal genetic testing will have on pregnant women and on their overall health. It is not yet even clear whether the testing that is already in place, AFP screening and chromosomal analysis for women aged 35 and older, is beneficial to women's health. Second, it is likely, at least for the foreseeable future, that the counseling available in physicians' offices will not meet the standard set for genetic counseling, adopted in order to ensure the benefits of genetic testing and to protect individuals from harm.

The next decades will bring a continued expansion in genetic technology and in the use of genetic testing in many areas of health care, including obstetrics. Certainly, most of the questions posed here cannot be answered until a large number of women actually go through the processes of considering testing and of the testing itself. One of the challenges faced is to offer testing in its initial stages in an investigative manner that both protects the women involved and allows important questions to be addressed. Ideally, new tests would be offered only in those settings where adequate counseling, follow-up, and safeguards are in place, and where a conscientious effort is made to answer difficult questions about the impact of testing on patients and their families.

Currently, concerns about the risk to a fetus of diagnostic methods such as amniocentesis and chorionic villi sampling are considered an understandable reason for a woman's decision to decline prenatal genetic testing. Those concerns also underlie policies limiting testing to older women or women with a specific genetic risk. Soon, however, it will be possible to perform genetic testing on fetal cells obtained by withdrawing blood from a pregnant woman's arm, eliminating the most obvious physical risk factor. The claim may then be made that there is no good reason not to have testing done. Widespread testing could potentially be initiated—and for all pregnant women. It is imperative both that solid evidence exists indicating that prenatal genetic testing is truly beneficial to the majority of women, and that effective mechanisms for reducing the burdens involved in testing are available before the routine testing of every pregnant woman becomes standard medical practice.

NOTES

Planned Parenthood v. Casey, 112 S. Ct. 2791 (1992).

BIBLIOGRAPHY

BEESON, D., & Golbus, M. S. (1979). Anxiety engendered by amniocentesis. *Birth Defects, 15*, 191–197.

BOSS, J. A. (1990). How voluntary prenatal diagnosis and selective abortion increase the abnormal human gene pool. *Birth, 17*, 75–79.

BOTKIN, J. R. (1988). The legal concept of wrongful life. *Journal of the American Medical Association, 259*, 1541–1545.

BOTKIN, J. R. (1990). Prenatal screening: Professional standards and the limits of parental choice. *Obstetrics and Gynecology, 75*, 875–880.

CACCIA, N., Johnson, J. M., Robinson, G. E., & Barna, T. (1991). Impact of prenatal testing on maternal-fetal bonding: Chorionic villus sampling versus amniocentesis. *American Journal of Obstetrics and Gynecology, 165*, 1122–1125.

CASSELL, E. (1977). The function of medicine. *Hastings Center Report, 7*, 16–19.

DIXSON, B., Richards, T. L., Reinsch, R. N., Edrich, B. S., Matson, M. R., & Jones, O. W. (1981). Mid-trimester amniocentesis: Subjective maternal responses. *Journal of Reproductive Medicine, 26*, 10–16.

DRUGAN, A., Greb, A., Johnson, M. P., Krivchenia E. L., Uhlmann, W. R., Moghissi, K. S., & Evans, M. I. (1990). Determinants of parental decisions to abort for chromosome abnormalities. *Prenatal Diagnosis, 10*, 483–490.

ELIAS, S., & Annas, G. J. (1987). Reproductive genetics and the law. *Chadago*: Year Book, 113–120.

EVANS, M., Bottoms, S. F., Carlucci, T., Grant, J., Belsky, R. L., Solyom, A. E., Quigg, M. H., & LaFerla, J. J. (1988). Determinants of altered anxiety after abnormal maternal serum alpha fetoprotein screening. *American Journal of Obstetrics and Gynecology, 159*, 1501–1504.

EVERS-KIEBOOMS, G., Swerts, A., & Van den Berghe, H. (1988). Psychological aspects of amniocentesis: Anxiety feelings in three different risk groups. *Clinical Genetics, 33*, 196–206.

FEENY, D., & Torrance, G. W. (1989). Incorporating utility-based quality of life assessment measures in clinical trials. *Medical Care, 27*, S190–S204.

FINLEY, S. C., Varner, P. D., Vinson, P. C., & Finley, W. H. (1977). Participants' reaction to amniocentesis and prenatal genetic studies. *Journal of the American Medical Association, 238*, 2377–2381.

FLETCHER, J. C., & Evans, M. I. (1983). Maternal bonding in early fetal ultrasound examinations. *New England Journal of Medicine, 308*, 392–393.

GATES, E. A. (1990). Maternal choice: Will it work both ways? *Women's Health Issues, 1*, 25–27.

HADDOW, J. E., Palomaki, G. E., Knight, G. J., Williams, J., Pulkkinen, A., Canick, J. A., Saller, D. N., & Bowers, G. B. (1992). Prenatal screening for Down's syndrome with use of maternal serum markers. *New England Journal of Medicine, 327*, 588–593.

HOLMES-SEIDEL, M., Ryynanen, M., & Lindenbaum, R. H. (1987). Parental decisions regarding termination of pregnancy following prenatal detection of sex chromosome anomalies. *Prenatal Diagnosis, 7*, 239–244.

HSIA, Y. E., & Hirschhorn, K. (1979). What is genetic counseling? In Y. E. Hsia, K. Hirschhorn, R. L. Silverberg, & L. Godmilow (Eds.), *Counseling in genetics* (pp. 1–29). New York: Alan R. Liss.

KEENAN, K. L., Basso, D., Goldkrand, J., & Butler, W. J. (1991). Low level of maternal serum alpha-fetoprotein: Its associated anxiety and the effects of genetic counseling. *American Journal of Obstetrics and Gynecology, 164*, 54–56.

KERSHNER, M. A., Hammond, E. A., & Donnenfeld, A. E. (1992). Knowledge of genetics among residents in obstetrics and gynecology. *American Journal of Human Genetics, 51*(S), A16.

LIPPMAN, A. (1991). Prenatal genetic testing and screening: Constructing needs and reinforcing inequities. *American Journal of Law and Medicine, 17*, 15–50.

LIU, A. N. (1987). Wrongful life: Some of the problems. *Journal of Medical Ethics, 13*, 69–73.

MARTEAU, T. M., Cook, R., Kidd, J., Michie, S., Johnston, M., Slack, J., & Shaw, R. W. (1992). The psychological effects of false positive results in prenatal screening for fetal abnormality: A prospective study. *Prenatal Diagnosis, 12*, 205–214.

MEYER, J. L., Edwards, J. G., Young, S. R., & Brooks, K. A. (1992). Human resource study on genetic counselors. *American Journal of Human Genetics, 51*(S), A269.

PHILLIPS, O. P., Elias, S., Shulman, L. P., Andersen, R. N., Morgan, C. D., & Simpson, J. L. (1992). Maternal serum screening for fetal Down syndrome in women less than 35 years of age using alpha-fetoprotein, hCG and unconjugated estriol: A prospective 2-year study. *Obstetrics and Gynecology, 80,* 353–358.

PHIPPS, S., & Zinn, A. B. (1986). Psychological responses to amniocentesis: Mood state and adaptation to pregnancy. *American Journal of Medical Genetics, 25,* 131–142.

RAPP, R. (1987). Moral pioneers: Women, men and fetuses on a frontier of reproductive technology. *Women and Health, 13,* 101–116.

ROBINSON, G. E., Garner, D. M., Olmsted, M. P., Shime, J., Hutton, E. M., & Crawford, B. M. (1988). Anxiety reduction after chorionic villus sampling and genetic amniocentesis. *American Journal of Obstetrics and Gynecology, 159,* 953–956.

ROTHMAN, B. K. (1986). *The tentative pregnancy.* New York: Penguin.

SHAW, M. W. (1984). Conditional prospective rights of the fetus. *Journal of Legal Medicine, 5,* 63–116.

SIMPSON, J. L. (1986). Genetic counseling and prenatal diagnosis. In S. G. Gabbe, J. R. Niebyl, & J. L. Simpson (Eds.), *Obstetrics: Normal and problem pregnancies* (pp. 211–244). New York: Churchill Livingstone.

SJOGREN, B., & Uddenberg, N. (1988). Decision making during the prenatal diagnostic procedure: A questionnaire and interview study of 211 women participating in prenatal diagnosis. *Prenatal Diagnosis, 8,* 263–273.

SPENCER, J. W., & Cox, D. N. (1988). A comparison of chorionic villi sampling and amniocentesis: Acceptability of procedure and maternal attachment to pregnancy. *Obstetrics and Gynecology, 72,* 714–778.

TABOR, A., & Jonsson, M. H. (1987). Psychological impact of amniocentesis on low risk women. *Prenatal Diagnosis, 7,* 443–449.

THOMPSON, L. (1989, October 10). The price of knowledge: Genetic tests that predict dire conditions become a two-edged sword. *Washington Post.*

WERTZ, D. C., Janes, S. R., Rosenfield, J. M., & Erbe, R. W. (1992). Attitudes toward the prenatal diagnosis of cystic fibrosis: Factors in decision making among affected families. *American Journal of Human Genetics, 50,* 1077–1085.

10 Collective Silences, Collective Fictions:

How Prenatal Diagnostic Testing Became Part of Routine Prenatal Care

NANCY ANNE PRESS AND
CAROLE H. BROWNER

Introduction

Prenatal diagnostic testing has entered a new realm. In the past decade it has ceased to be defined and delimited by amniocentesis, an invasive procedure offered only to women considered to be at particular risk for bearing a child with a birth defect. Instead, with the advent of population-based, rather than risk-based screening, prenatal testing for the detection of birth defects has joined the routine modes of scrutiny to which women's pregnancies are increasingly subjected. This has occurred with little explicit comment on the profound change it represents. Yet today, in many areas of the United States and Europe, every pregnant woman is considered eligible for prenatal diagnostic screening. This not only effectively marks every pregnancy as potentially "at risk," but places in the path of every pregnant woman the possibility of facing a decision about the continuation or termination of her pregnancy based on the presence of a birth anomaly. What this large group of "low risk" pregnant women think about such population-based screening and how they make decisions about participating in or opting out of it has been little investigated. The purpose of this chapter is to explore those questions. In doing so, we will also attempt to discover how this major development in the management of pregnancy has been effected with such silence and such ease.

The paradigmatic case in the development and expansion of population-based prenatal screening is the maternal serum alpha-fetoprotein (AFP) test. It was originally designed to screen a pregnant woman's blood for indications in the fetus of neural tube defects, which are serious malformations of the brain and spine.[1] Currently this technology is being expanded to include further analyses from the same maternal blood sample. This "triple marker" analysis will make the test nearly as effective a screen for chromosomal abnormalities, including Down syndrome, as it is for neural tube defects.[2] Throughout the United States today approximately 65% of women enrolled in prenatal care are already being screened for AFP levels (Meaney, Riggle, & Cunningham, 1993), and the Department of Health and Human Services recently made it a goal of their Healthy People 2000 initiative to "increase to at least 90 percent the proportion of women . . . who are offered screening and counseling on prenatal detection of fetal abnormalities" (USDHHS, 1991). In California that goal is closest to realization, since there is a legal mandate in the state that health care providers offer AFP screening to all pregnant women as part of routine prenatal care. The California State program, therefore, provides an excellent opportunity to examine how the institutionalization of AFP screening is perceived and reacted to by the women who are its consumers.[3]

The research on which this chapter is based was undertaken in part to assess the role of cultural differences in women's decisions about whether or not to participate in the California AFP program. We interviewed women with different ethnic and social-class backgrounds and degrees of religiosity because we believed that these characteristics would influence test acceptance. Contrary to our expectations, not only did the overwhelming majority agree to be tested, but they showed marked similarities in the reasoning behind their decisions.

We believe this unanticipated result occurred because women's understandings about the AFP test were shaped primarily by the way the test was described to them by their health care providers and in a booklet prepared by the state's AFP program. We suggest that the structure and content of this information increased test acceptability far more than it succeeded in increasing knowledge about the test. The strength of this effect may even explain the absence in our sample of the class and ethnic differences suggested by previous literature on women's use of reproductive genetic testing (Rapp, 1988).

It would be wrong, however, to conclude that this absence of variation along class and ethnic lines demonstrates the insignificance of cultural factors in decisions about the AFP test. Rather, we believe it demonstrates that there exist a set of cultural beliefs, understandings, and values, shared by those who offered and those who accepted AFP screening, which enhanced the acceptability of the test. Central among these is a fundamental faith in the power and value of scientific knowledge and the solutions science provides. In pregnancy, this view is expressed in the belief that undergoing routine prenatal care will help lead to a healthy birth. Yet in the arena of prenatal diagnostic testing, this optimistic faith must coexist with the more ominous themes of serious birth anomalies, selective abortion, and eugenic selection that prenatal diagnostic testing by definition entails. These contradictions create a tension which makes health care professionals uncomfortable discussing, and women uncomfortable contemplating, the realities of AFP screening. Our data suggest that this tension is reduced through the creation of a collective fiction: the presentation of AFP screening as a simple and routine part of prenatal care. We will demonstrate that this fiction is effective because it serves the interests of all parties involved. It serves the state public health program's purpose of trying to reduce the incidence of neural tube defects, health care providers' desire to limit their legal liability, and women's complex needs to be reassured about the outcome of their pregnancy and to leave open but uncontemplated the option of terminating an affected pregnancy.

Research Design

This analysis is based on data collected from the pilot phase of a longer-term study.[4] The pilot sample comprised 40 Catholic, pregnant women, between the ages of 20 and 34, all of whom had begun prenatal medical care before their 20th week of pregnancy.[5] We chose to work only with women raised Catholic for the pilot study. We speculated that, because of their church's objection to abortion, these women might be more likely than others to hold developed opinions on the subject of prenatal diagnostic testing.

One-half of the total sample was Mexican-American and one-half non-Hispanic white;[6] one-half were from middle-class and one-half from lower-class backgrounds.[7] All were patients at one of three sites of a single health maintenance organization (HMO) in Southern California.[8] All had either received a negative AFP result (n = 36)[9] or had refused the screening test (n = 4).

Data were obtained during semi-structured interviews and by observing the prenatal intake in which women were told about the AFP program by nursing staff. Interviews with informants took place at approximately their 24th week of pregnancy, when all prenatal diagnostic test results would have been received and all decisions based on those results made. For most informants this was about two months after being given information about the AFP program.

We also interviewed the clinic administrators and the nursing staff who conducted prenatal intakes at each of the three field sites, as well as an opportunistic sample of Southern Californian physicians and other health care providers, on issues surrounding AFP screening and prenatal diagnostic testing in general.

The Medicolegal Context of the California AFP Program

When the State of California created an AFP program, it included an elaborate informed consent and refusal process in keeping with the view of bioethicists that "participants in prenatal screening programs should understand the nature and purpose of the screening" (Faden et al., 1985). Ironically, in making this test standard-of-care for pregnant women, a legal liability was created for providers which may work against the very goals of informed consent outlined by bioethicists. The possibility of lost paperwork or later claims of inadequate test explanation present great legal and financial risk for providers. In contrast, the test procedure—a blood draw from the pregnant woman's arm—carries virtually no physical risk for the patient. Therefore, in weighing the costs and benefits of AFP screening for their patients and themselves, providers may conclude that the most expedient route is to encourage women to accept the test.

In fact, many providers we interviewed, both at the HMO and elsewhere, raised concerns about legal liability in discussing AFP screening, stating that their fear of legal ramifications influenced what they told their patients about the AFP program. Several claimed that the State's mandate to offer AFP screening was, in medicolegal terms, tantamount to a requirement that they test all their pregnant patients. Some even admitted that they make it difficult for a woman to refuse testing. One said, "I just tell them, 'Take it.'" Even physicians who are more willing to accept no for an answer may feel a need to bring the topic up several times simply to be able to chart a patient's repeated refusals. Women, who most likely have no idea what is motivating their health care provider, may as a result perceive this test as something very important.

The same concerns led those in charge at the HMO where we worked to create careful protocols to ensure staff cooperation in meeting the State's requirement that all pregnant women be informed about the AFP program. At one site, memos stamped with the slogan "Think AFP" urged providers to develop "an AFP consciousness"; at another, the lab technician had a special calendar file which alerted him when a patient was nearing the end of the time when she was eligible for the screening test. The third site employed a special monitor among whose functions it was to phone women who had missed scheduled AFP appointments in order to address any reservations they might have about the test. Thus, for example, women who expressed reservations about the test because they would not terminate a pregnancy for any reason were categorized as having misinformation and told about other reasons to undergo AFP screening, such as advance delivery room preparation, were a problem to be uncovered. In cases such as these, the distinction between informing women and persuading them seemed blurred, and is likely to have contributed to the high rates of AFP acceptance we observed.[10]

What Women Were Told about the AFP Test by Their Health Care Providers

A content analysis of the 40 prenatal intakes we observed strongly reinforced the view that the HMO's de facto definition of AFP "compliance" was the obtaining of agreement to be tested, not simply the provision of information to aid decision-making.

While, as a rule, the prenatal intakes lasted from 15 to 30 minutes, no more than two minutes was ever devoted to discussion of the AFP test. Nearly all the information provided concerned the test procedure itself and what a woman had to do to obtain testing. Consent was thereby implicitly assumed unless a patient explicitly indicated that her wishes were to the contrary. Moreover, AFP screening was generally introduced in the part of the intake in which other blood work was scheduled. Since these other blood tests were presented as routine, but not voluntary, the effect was to routinize the AFP test as part of the HMO's standard prenatal care package.

The specific language used by nursing staff to introduce and describe AFP could also be seen to further the goal of test acceptance by means of routinization. Thus, the frequent use of phrases such as, "It's just a simple blood test," "It's only a prick in your arm," or "It won't hurt you or the baby" seemed intended to diminish test apprehension. In contrast, statements such as, "This is our AFP program, the government screening here in California," "We do recommend the test for everyone, though you have the option not to have it done," and "It's not mandatory, but it is recommended" seemed geared more toward direct persuasion. Women were sometimes asked if they had any questions. They almost never did. Nothing was done to help them formulate such questions, and the prior conversational flow, in which the nurse had asked the questions while the patient answered, may have led our informants to feel that a question would be an imposition. The rushed nurses never probed past an initial patient response of "I have no questions."

Perhaps even more striking than the form and content of the information women received about the AFP program is what they were not told. The conditions for which AFP screens, for example, were at best defined vaguely as "misgrowths of the brain or spine" or merely glossed by phrases such as "the test looks for some birth defects in the baby" or "the test shows how your baby is developing."[11] In no intake was a woman given information about the physiological, emotional, or familial effects of any of these conditions, nor were the kinds of decisions a woman would face in the event of a positive diagnosis ever discussed; the words "abortion" or "pregnancy termination" were mentioned only twice during all 40 intakes. Our view that this was not an accidental omission is supported by the following comment from a nurse who had important health education responsibilities at one site:

> Once . . . I said that if there was a problem [with the AFP] it was then up to the woman to decide whether to continue the pregnancy or not. Later [my supervisor] told me never to talk about that because . . . [she has seen that] when she says anything about pregnancy termination, the women stiffen. So now I'm real careful and never mention pregnancy termination when I'm telling them about the AFP test.

In sum, in our provider interviews and prenatal observations we found both that a tension existed between the ethical objective that pregnant women be permitted to fully consider the implications of prenatal testing and the legal injunction that providers offer women the test, and that providers responded to this tension by blurring the line between informing and persuading. We would also suggest, however, that providers could rest assured in the belief that women did not want to hear more, a belief that could be supported by the observation that women neither asked many questions nor seemed resistant to the idea of being tested. Health care providers also knew that all these women would have another source of information about the AFP test.

The AFP Booklet—Another Source of Information

All health care providers are required to give their prenatal patients a booklet prepared by the State of California that describes the AFP program. The "California Alpha-Fetoprotein Screening Program" booklet (State of California, 1988) was written to be comprehensible to anyone reading at a tenth-grade level (Lustig, Linda, personal communication, 1991). In our view, however, the text is quite dense and difficult, often providing both more and less information than would seem necessary. In this regard, the booklet's discussion of the meaning of positive test results is instructive in the light of data we will present below on our informants' particularly poor understanding of this point.

One-half of page two of the booklet is devoted to a detailed chart of the various reasons why a woman might receive a positive AFP test result. Yet the booklet never defines a positive test result as a negative event, and it requires some sophistication in medical language to be aware of this counterintuitive usage of the word "positive."

In addition, descriptions of some of the situations that might lead to a positive test result are accurate without being particularly informative. For instance, "normal variation of the AFP level" is listed as the second most likely cause of a positive result raising, for some informants, questions about how test results could be definitively interpreted.

Moreover, in describing the conditions for which the test was designed to screen, the wording is surprisingly vague. Compare, for example, the straightforward syntax of "there may be twins" to the complex and hedging quality of "additional tests may be needed to find out if this [result] is due to birth defects such as neural tube defects or abdominal wall defects." Since additional tests are also needed to ascertain the presence of twins, the most reasonable explanation for this syntactic change is a desire to divert attention from the realm of possible birth anomalies and the choices they might entail to the more routine domain of "further testing."

But, should one conclude that the AFP booklet is simply an example of poorly written patient information materials, consider that nowhere in its pages is there a clear statement that this is a test to find out if a baby will be born with medical problems of so severe a nature that a parent might consider them incompatible with a decent life; neither is it mentioned that there is no treatment for the great majority of these conditions other than ending the pregnancy. In fact, it is not until the very last page of text that one finds a small section entitled "What happens if the tests show that the fetus has a birth defect?" The reply is that further information would be provided on the defect and its effects, that "different options will be discussed," and that services are available to "support whatever decision the woman makes." "Option" and "decision," therefore, appear to be code words for abortion, while "special services" and "support" are the only indications that this decision may be painful or morally difficult. We contend that the obscurity of this language, and the out-of-the-way placement of the paragraph, are in keeping with the tone of the entire booklet. Thus while the AFP test raises alarming possibilities and disturbing solutions, the booklet is written in a way that obscures and reassures rather than informs.[12] In the section below, we will examine the consequences of these various silences and omissions in the process of informing women about AFP testing.

What Women Knew about the AFP Test

The flaws in the procedures for informing pregnant women about the AFP screening test were best revealed when we assessed women's level of AFP knowledge after they had accepted or refused the screening test.[13] We did this by developing a series of questions based on the AFP informed consent/refusal form. The points which women aver to have understood in signing the form are as follows: (1) the names of conditions AFP screening can detect; (2) the effects of those conditions on children and adults; (3) what next steps would be suggested if they received a positive result; (4) that the test is voluntary.

Ninety percent of our informants stated that they remembered getting this booklet and 75% said that they had read and understood it. We found, however, that they remembered little of the information it contained. Most notably, not one could explain adequately what were the various conditions that might yield a positive test result. Only 30% of informants recognized the term neural tube defect and of those who did, two-thirds had no accurate idea of what a neural tube defect was, several confusing it with an ectopic or "tubal" pregnancy. The term spina bifida had a 60% name recognition but only about one-half of those informants felt they could define the condition. The majority who did so seemed to be taking a guess based on the name, such as, "Wouldn't it be a spinal disease?" Only 10% had any idea about the symptoms and consequences of spina bifida and all who did had personal knowledge of some-one with the condition. Fewer than one-half knew what their doctor would want to do next if their test result proved positive. Finally, more than one-third incorrectly thought or suspected that pregnant women were required by the state to take the AFP test.

What Our Informants Want to Know

Yet neither the way women were told about the test by their health care providers, nor the manner in which the official state booklet is written, provides a full explanation of our infor-mants' simultaneously high rates of test acceptance and low lev-els of test comprehension. To these factors must be added what the women themselves said they wanted to know about the test. For if the state and the health care providers have reasons for wishing to present AFP screening within an idiom of routine prenatal care, our data reveal that our informants share this preference and were able, therefore, to accept this "simple" blood test without feeling the need to understand very much about it or ponder its implications. Thus, even after women's lack of AFP knowledge was revealed to them through our ques-tioning, they overwhelmingly professed satisfaction with the amount of AFP information they had been given.

Informants' responses were notably brief and stereotypical to all interview questions which concerned either the moral as-pects of prenatal diagnostic testing, their reasons for test accep-tance, or what they might do following a hypothetical positive result. This contrasted with their lengthy and detailed replies to questions during the rest of the interview. We also found that the words "abortion" or "pregnancy termination" were rarely uttered by a woman in answering these questions unless and until the interviewer used them. This suggested to us something close to a cultural taboo on open discussion and careful consideration of just those issues bioethicists see as most germane to decisions and understandings about prenatal testing.

Precisely because women appeared to have difficulty articulating their own views about the ethics of prenatal diagnostic testing, we developed three short scenarios that represented major bioethical stances on the subject. The "Disabilities Rights" scenario used the voice of a handicapped woman who expressed the fear that had the AFP test existed when her own mother was pregnant, she might not be alive today. The "Religious Fundamentalist" scenario expressed an objection to prenatal tests because they can tempt humans into making Godlike decisions about who is "entitled" to life. Placed between the two was a "Pro-Testing" scenario told from the perspective of the parents of a handicapped child. They discussed the difficulties and stress of life for a handicapped child and its family and expressed wholehearted approval of prenatal diagnostic testing because it can help avert such births and allow couples to "try again."

We anticipated that women would find two of the three positions mutually exclusive, and that most would identify at least one as reflecting their own point of view. We were surprised, therefore, to find that the great majority (80%) could endorse none of these positions. The reason appeared to be that most informants simultaneously supported testing while opposing abortion. Thus, while the assumption underlying all three scenarios was that a positive test result would lead to terminating the pregnancy, our informants did not appear to see a necessary link between these two events. Many informants, for example, agreed with the Religious Fundamentalist position that parents should let God decide who would and would not be born and which stated that a negative aspect of prenatal diagnostic tests was that they could "tempt" some parents to intervene. But they did not regard this temptation as a sufficient reason not to make the tests available. In explanation they stated that although others might use test results as a basis for pregnancy termination, they themselves would never do so.

The majority of our informants seemed impatient with the question about the moral correctness of *offering* prenatal diagnostic testing with which we ended each scenario. In fact,

hardly a single informant could endorse any suggestion that offering prenatal diagnostic testing was negative, or even problematic. Yet they consistently framed their scenario responses to
answer a question we had not asked: How should one judge a
woman who terminated a pregnancy following a positive prenatal test result? Often informants' responses to all three scenarios constituted a single, connected consideration of this unasked
question. They emphasized the necessity for individual choice
and refused to criticize a woman faced with this difficult decision. Thus, the most frequently repeated statements were, "It's
her decision," "It's up to the individual," "You can't say for
someone else."

It is plausible that these responses are an artifact of our all-
Catholic study population. However, we find it more likely that
they reflect deep contradictions within these women's belief systems regarding the selective abortion of anomalous fetuses, and
that those contradictions are shared by much of the general
population. This view is supported by our informants' responses to a standardized measure we devised to elicit hypothetical willingness to terminate a pregnancy for certain congenital conditions.[14] Analysis of these data reveal that close to
70% of our informants believed that they would definitely or
probably terminate a pregnancy for at least some of these conditions. Significantly, the most frequently selected conditions
were those for which AFP screens. This is not out of line with
California state statistics which indicate that approximately
80% of all California women who receive a confirmed positive
AFP test result for nonremediable conditions choose to terminate their pregnancies (Genetic Disease Branch, 1990).

Why Women Want the AFP Screening Test

When asked what they liked about the AFP test and why they
had agreed to be tested, the possibility of being able to end a
pregnancy was mentioned extremely rarely. The most frequent
response was that the test could offer reassurance that their
pregnancy was going well. We have written elsewhere that
many women consider prenatal medical care to be a "ritual of
reassurance" (Browner & Press, 1991) rather than an opportu-

nity to receive specific services or safeguards. Studies of other prenatal diagnostic tests have found that reassurance is also a prime reason women seek such testing (Marteau et al., 1989; Green, 1990; Nielsen, 1981; Rothman, 1986). However, specific statements made by informants also suggest that many believed that the AFP test would not only *assure* but also *ensure* their baby's health. Thus, women frequently stated that they had accepted the AFP test "Just to be safe." Others stated that they took the test "because I wanted to make sure my baby would be the healthiest that it could be," or "I wanted to do anything that could help me or my baby." This last response expresses with particular clarity the ambiguity involved in a screening program, offered as a routine part of maternal prenatal health care, that can diagnose but for the most part not cure the conditions it detects.

The second most common reason women said they took the test was that it would provide them with "knowledge." Much has been written about the extreme salience of scientific knowledge in Western society.[15] Some of that literature suggests that information which cannot prevent harm or provide an acceptable path for action might not constitute valuable knowledge. But such views were not shared by our informants who appeared to believe that scientific information offered to them could not, or should not, be refused. Rather they repeatedly expressed the belief that "the more you know about your child the better off you are" and wondered "how could it hurt to know?" This was true even though the majority of informants knew or feared that nothing could be done medically if the fetus were found to have a problem and, as we have stated above, in the main denied that they would use knowledge derived from prenatal testing as a basis for action.

Conclusion

Both the California state AFP program and health care providers present AFP screening as an uncomplicated and routine part of prenatal care. In doing so, they place it firmly under the rubric of broadly shared, contemporary American cultural beliefs about the value of scientific knowledge and medical care.

At the same time, this presentation enables all concerned in offering and accepting AFP testing to remain silent about issues on which there is no societal consensus—such as the appropriateness of aborting fetal anomalies and the eugenic implications of the practice.

This selective perception of what issues constitute the arena of prenatal testing is not imposed upon women. Rather, it fits within their own understandings and serves their own desire to avoid the discussion, if not the use, of pregnancy termination. It is precisely for these reasons that these silences and fictions should be seen as collective. The question that remains is whether this is an appropriate way to create policy and action in a society faced with increasingly acrimonious legislative and societal debate over abortion, growing pressure to make medical decisions deemed "cost-effective," and the rapidly accelerating capacity to discover medical problems in fetuses long before their birth.

ACKNOWLEDGMENTS

The research was supported in part by NICHD Grant #HD11944, with additional funding from the UCLA Academic Senate and the UCLA Chicano Studies Research Center. We gratefully thank Richard Carroll, Jan Simpson, and Arthur J. Rubel for their helpful comments on earlier drafts of this paper. We also wish to thank the Genetics Disease Branch of the California State Department of Health Services for their gracious cooperation, as well as the HMO where we collected our data for their very generous contributions of time, access to patients, and overall support of the research.

NOTES

1. The most common neural tube defects are anencephaly, an absence of skull and brain, which is always fatal, and spina bifida, a failure of the spinal column to close, which produces symptoms of widely varying severity. Neural tube defects are among the most common birth defects. In California the prevalence rate is approximately 1:1,000 live births (Greenberg, James, & Oakley, 1983).
2. AFP screening alone detects close to 90% of cases of anencephaly and somewhat over two-thirds of open and closed spina bifida. Through the addition of analyses of unconjugated estriol and chorionic gonadotropin, the other two components of the triple marker screening, about 60% of Down syndrome can be detected.
3. Please note that our intent here is not to critique the California AFP program per se. Rather, we offer this analysis in the hope that it pro-

vides insight into both the implementation of one particular prenatal screening program and the broader issues surrounding the implementation of programs of this type.

4. Because the results reported here are based on data obtained from a relatively small number of women, any generalizations should, of course, be made with caution. However, preliminary analysis of the 125 additional cases from our main study, which includes a broader range of demographics, appears to support the analysis presented here.

5. Blood must be drawn for the AFP test between the 15th and 20th weeks of gestation. Thus, women who present themselves for their first prenatal medical appointment after their 20th week cannot be offered the test.

6. A woman was considered non–Hispanic white if she and her parents had been born in the United States and none of her grandparents had been born in any Latin American country. She was considered Mexican-American if she, either of her parents, or any of her grandparents had been born in Mexico, as long as the informant herself had come to the United States before the age of ten. The criteria for those two categories, therefore, are not strictly parallel. They imply a longer and more vigorous connection with the country of family origin for Mexican Americans than for other immigrant groups, and are based on the observations of researchers familiar with the Los Angeles Mexican-American community (Gilbert, Jean, personal communication, 1989; Hayes-Bautista, David, personal communication, 1990). Informants' self-ascribed ethnicity was consistent with these definitions.

7. We used mode of payment for medical services as a heuristic device to define our middle-class and lower-class samples. Thus, those women whose medical services at the HMO were paid for by MediCal (the California Medicaid system) were considered lower class; those whose services were subsidized by their employers were considered middle class. During the interview, we collected additional sociodemographic information, including income and educational level. We found that our heuristic did produce two distinct groups: Household income was just over $11,000 for the MediCal group and $43,000 for the middle-class group. Close to 60% of the MediCal recipients had not graduated high school; in contrast, just one middle-class informant had not graduated high school and over 40% had received at least some post-high school training.

8. Because this HMO has a MediCal contract with the State of California, we were able to recruit women from both SES groups from the same facilities. We believe that this has important methodological advantages. We believe that it is often impossible to separate reported class differences in, for example, patient compliance, from the differences in health care delivery provided lower-class and middle-class patients. In this case, however, we could observe that all women received identical services.

9. Three women in the sample received an initial positive test result that was reinterpreted as negative after ultrasound corrected the gestational age of the fetus.

10. Rates of AFP acceptance in California vary sharply by patient population and health care setting. Aggregate statewide statistics indicate a 60% acceptance rate. However, an early study by Richwald (1989) found that only 34% of low SES patients in seven Los Angeles County clinics agreed to the procedure when they had to pay for it themselves. (MediCal now covers the costs of the test.) In contrast, some private physicians report that close to 100% of their patients undergo AFP screening. Our own informal survey of other HMOs in Southern California yielded acceptance rates of around 85%, which is similar to those at our field sites.

11. HMO policy dictated that Down syndrome not be mentioned by staff in regard to AFP testing because HMO management was skeptical about the accuracy of AFP test results for this disorder.

12. The political motivations for this type of presentation are not hard to find. According to sources close to the creation of the California program, legislative approval was constantly in doubt. Eventual success has been attributed to a strategy that kept the program's profile as low as possible by splitting the bill into regulations approved in committee and funding included in the state's annual budget. Even so, this author was told that "the legislation got through by the skin of its teeth . . . [because] anything today that involves the 'A' word is hot."

13. Few studies have been done to assess participants' level of knowledge about AFP screening (but see Faden et al. [1985], Marteau et al. [1989], and Green [1988]), and only work by Faden et al. (1989) represents a detailed study of how well women understood the information that they received about the test. Although Faden's data are not completely comparable with ours, she also found "substantial gaps in the knowledge base of women" who had undergone AFP testing (p. 1382).

14. Attitudes concerning various handicaps and developmental disabilities were assessed through the Developmental Disabilities Attitudes Measure (DDAM), a ranking device developed by the researchers. This four-point Likert Scale comprised two sorting tasks. The symptoms of 18 conditions that are genetically transmitted were listed on cards. Informants were first asked to sort the cards according to their degree of concern about the birth of a child with each symptom. They were then asked to re-sort the cards according to how likely they thought they would be to terminate a pregnancy for each symptom.

15. See Habermas (1972), Bleier (1984), Wright and Treacher (1982), Reiser (1978), and Rose (1976).

BIBLIOGRAPHY

BLEIER, R. (1984). *Science and gender: A critique of biology and its theories on women.* New York: Pergamon Press.

BROWNER, C. H., & Press, N. A. (1991). The normalization of prenatal screening: Women's acquiescence to the alpha fetoprotein blood test [Paper presented in Wenner-Gren Symposium #113, "The Politics of Reproduction" Teresópolis, Brazil].

FADEN, R. R., Chwalow, A. J., Ovel-Crosby, E., et al. (1985). What participants understand about a maternal serum alpha-fetoprotein screening program. *American Journal of Public Health, 75*, 1381–1384.

GENETIC Disease Branch. (1990, March). A report to the legislature. *Review of Current Genetics Programs.* Berkeley, CA: California Department of Health Services.

GREEN, D. (1988). Maternal anxiety and perception of benefit from the California maternal serum alpha fetoprotein screening program [Unpublished Master's Thesis]. University of California, Irvine.

GREEN, J. M. (1990). Calming or harming? A critical review of psychological effects of fetal diagnosis on pregnant women. *Galton Institute Occasional Papers*, Second Series, No. 2.

GREENBERG, F., James, L. M., & Oakley, G. P. (1983). Estimates of birth prevalence rates of spina bifida in the United States from computer generated maps. *American Journal of Obstetrics and Gynecology, 145*, 570–573.

HABERMAS, J. (1972). *Knowledge and human interests.* London: Heinemann.

MARTEAU, T., Johnstone, M., Shaw, R. W., Michie, S., Kidd, J., & New, M. (1989). The impact of prenatal screening and diagnostic testing upon the cognitions, emotions, and behaviour of pregnant women. *Journal of Psychosomatic Research, 33*, 7–16.

MEANEY, J. F., Riggle, S. M., & Cunningham, G. C. (1993). Providers and consumers of prenatal genetic services: What do the data tell us? *Fetal Diagnosis and Therapy, 8*(Suppl. 1), pp. 18–27.

NIELSEN, C. C. (1981). An encounter with modern medical technology: Women's experiences with amniocentesis. *Women and Health, 6*, 109–124.

RAPP, R. (1988). Chromosomes and communication: The discourse of genetic counseling. *Medical Anthropology Quarterly New Series, 2*(2), 143–157.

REISER, S. J. (1978). *Medicine and the reign of technology.* Cambridge: Cambridge University Press.

RICHWALD, G., Friedland, J., Nelson, A., & Silberman, I. (1989). Evaluation of maternal serum alpha-fetoprotein screening in public clinics in Los Angeles County, California.

ROSE, H., & Rose, S. (Eds.). (1976). *The Ideology of/in the Natural Sciences.* Boston: Schenkman.

ROTHMAN, B. K. (1986). *The tentative pregnancy: Prenatal diagnosis and the future of motherhood.* New York: Penguin.

STATE of California Department of Health Services, Genetic Disease Branch. (1988). *The California Alpha Fetoprotein Screening Program*. Berkeley, CA.

UNITED States Department of Health and Human Services. (1991). Healthy people 2000: National health promotion and disease prevention objective. In *Fall Report*, (Publication No. 91–50212, pp. 382–383). Washington, DC: USDHHS.

WRIGHT, P., & Treacher, A. (1982). *The problem of medical knowledge: Examining the social construction of medicine*. Edinburgh: Edinburgh University Press.

Women's Responses to Prenatal Diagnosis:

A Sociocultural Perspective on Diversity

RAYNA RAPP

Introduction

The technology of amniocentesis was first developed experimentally from the late 1960s forward with and for women who were at high risk of transmitting chromosomal and genetic disorders. It quickly spread during the 1970s and 1980s to those sectors of the American population who had access to both the knowledge and payment plans that sanctioned its use, that is, overwhelmingly, the middle classes (Cowan, 1992, 1993; McDonough, 1990). Now another kind of experimentation and routinization of prenatal diagnostic technology is under way as women from much less privileged backgrounds gain access to the test and, increasingly, opt to use it (Hsu, 1989; MHRA, 1990).

For the past nine years I have been studying the social impact and cultural meaning of this "second wave" of amniocentesis in New York City, where the test is widely available to, and widely used by, women from diverse racial, ethnic, religious, and socioeconomic backgrounds. As a medical anthropologist, I am particularly interested in how this piece of reproductive technology intersects American cultural values in all their diverse complexity. Now New York City is not New Guinea, and prenatal diagnosis is not a secret initiation ritual. Nonetheless, standard anthropological methods of participant–observation

have enabled me to build a multilayered understanding of amniocentesis.

Working in a range of New York City hospitals, I have
watched more than 300 intake interviews with pregnant women
from culturally diverse backgrounds who are potential candidates for the test, trying to understand their questions, silences,
and responses to the information genetic counselors give them.
I have also interviewed more than 60 women (and 15 men) at
home after they have had the test to see what they thought
about it, and scores who refused to have the test, to find out
why a "routinizing technology" doesn't always stay on route.
Thirty-five genetic counselors and ten geneticists spoke with
me about the cultural diversity of their patients' backgrounds
and about their own attitudes on prenatal testing, disabilities,
and their variance in responses to the testing. An internship at
the city lab revealed something of how technicians think about
their work, while families in a support group for parents whose
children have Down syndrome helped me to understand the difference between a medical and a social definition of a chromosomal disability. In studying so many overlapping layers, I hope
to understand how women from diverse backgrounds experience the benefits and burdens of prenatal diagnosis, and to examine the problem of scientific literacy in general, and what
genetic testing means in specific, in a multicultural society.

The Research

I began my research by working out of the Prenatal Diagnosis
Laboratory (the PDL), set up by the Health Department of New
York City in 1978 explicitly to provide outreach to the urban
poor. The PDL is the largest cytogenetics lab attached to a public health facility in the United States. Its three to five genetic
counselors are circuit riders, servicing both private (that is,
middle-class) and clinic (that is, working-poor) patients in five
to seven hospitals, and its laboratory analyzes amniotic fluids
for 24 municipal hospitals. The population served by the lab
is about one-third African-American, one-third Hispanic, and
one-third white. But we should be cautious about such census
categories. Recent Haitian immigrants coming from the society

with the poorest medical services in the Western hemisphere are lumped together with native New Yorkers whose families have been in this country many generations longer than my own under the category "African-American"; the "old migrants" from Puerto Rico and the Dominican Republic end up in the same census box as recently arrived, war-torn Salvadorans and Nicaraguans, and middle-class Argentineans and Colombians. And the exotic "white" race includes Polish, Italian, and Irish Catholics; Ashkenazic and Sephardic Jews; Greek and Russian Orthodox; Pentecostalists; and Anglican Protestants as if they were a unified racial group by dint of not belonging to the minorities under surveillance.

In other words, "race" glosses a constantly expanding inventory of differences, and the salience of those differences change as the populations who come to the city and raise their families there evolve. But the historical and contemporary complexity of New York's fluid racial-ethnic map is often erased by the very categories of "difference" we are given. It is too easy to flatten this diversity into census boxes, each overgeneralized ethnic or racial group corresponding to a new stereotype. The same caveats apply to my more recent observations at Beth Israel Medical Center, where I am particularly interested in filling out my sample by observing working-class and lower middle-class patients sent for genetic services by the Hospital Insurance Plan (HIP), New York's oldest HMO. Beth Israel, too, serves a richly multilingual, multicultural patient population, approximately seven percent of whom are drawn from New York's Chinatown.

Findings

As an anthropologist, I am particularly interested in how issues of cultural diversity affect the range of responses to being offered an amniocentesis. But what I have found is that among New York's richly multicultural patient population sent for genetic counseling, women's access (or lack of access) to prenatal services where they are treated with respect and care influences their responses to prenatal testing far more than any specific cultural factor. That is, a woman's socioeconomic class standing, especially as it determines the neighborhoods in which she and her family live, and the areas surrounding the hospitals that will serve them, has already shaped prior health care experiences and the feelings of trust or mistrust with which a pregnant woman undertakes a counseling appointment. A woman's comfort or discomfort with the scientific worldview and scientific language is also deeply affected by her class-based experiences, especially, but not exclusively, through education. While the stories people told me about their aspirations, beliefs, and practices during pregnancy are clearly marked by concrete cultural legacies, these legacies are deeply intertwined with experiences more broadly shaped by class differences. This interplay of ethnocultural and class resources is easily illustrated in the reasons women give for accepting or rejecting an amniocentesis.

It is an axiom of genetic counseling that middle-class patients (disproportionately white) usually accept the test while poorer women (disproportionately from ethnic-racial minorities) are more likely to refuse it. But that generalization needs to be analyzed. Private patients are likely to have prior knowledge about the test and to have already made up their minds to use it by the time they come for genetic counseling. They will not make a counseling appointment unless they are already determined to have the test. Refusers in this class thus rarely get counted. But among clinic patients, an appointment with the genetic counselor may be the first opportunity they have to ponder the significance, risks, and benefits of prenatal testing. They then make up their minds in a context in which their decisions become part of hospital statistics.

Moreover, many African-American and Hispanic women *do* accept the test. Refusal rates vary dramatically from hospital to hospital. At one city hospital where the clinic serves in majority a Spanish-speaking low-income population, acceptance rates are high: 70–80%. At another, with an Afro-Caribbean and Spanish-speaking population, acceptance rates are low: 30–40% (Hsu, 1989). We could go fishing for a cultural explanation about pregnancy beliefs, medical attitudes, and so on. But a more simple observation is this: The first prenatal clinic is a stable and welcoming environment; women tend to be very comfortable there and tend to trust the nurses. By the time they arrive for an appointment with a genetic counselor, they have usually talked with a favorite nurse, often in Spanish, and feel competent to accept or reject the test.

In contrast, the second hospital has been a site of struggle over services for many years, and the prenatal clinic is a difficult environment in which to receive health care. Women (and often their young children) feel imprisoned in uncomfortable waiting rooms where they routinely spend two to three hours before being seen. By then the level of anger and frustration, exacerbated by the lack of communication, makes it much more likely that a woman will break a counseling appointment or sit through it in a state of distrust. Far more than simply "ethnic differences" are at stake in the microsociology of access to adequate and helpful medical services, and those various influences then condition acceptance rates.

The culturally specific, historical legacies of different communities also influence acceptance or rejection of the test. Such influences are neither simple nor straightforward, for they are deeply embedded in many collective histories of social, not just individual medical, risk. When I interviewed a 36-year-old Honduran UPS package inspector in a run-down neighborhood of Queens, for example, she seemed to have accepted an amniocentesis without great introspection. As the mother of two teenaged boys from a former marriage, she "just wanted everything to be all right." During the course of an hour's home interview, my tape was filled with her disinterested answers, interrupted by the flamboyant and sonorous testimony of her fervently Pentecostalist husband. He described his vivid visions of the infant Jesus protecting his own infant-to-be, swore that the prayers of his co-congregants had already healed all manner of potential problems the child might have faced, and used the occasion of my visit to witness the benefits of faith. He testified that Jesus had already cured fetal dim vision and a hole in the heart, two problems whose eschatology is central to both the Bible and discussions of birth defects. It was a stunning performance.

Later, Mari-Carmen walked me back to the subway, and without the pressures of husband or tape recorder told me that Pentecostalism was saving her husband, who had twice been

jailed on drug charges, and from whom she had separated because of his infidelities. Her chief worries centered on her older
sons, both having problems in school, one involved with a
neighborhood gang. If "having a baby for him" would stabilize
the family, she would accept the pregnancy, and the amniocentesis, and any other advice the doctor gave her, just as she had
accepted the Pentecostalist congregation. Without the benefit of
this shadow interview, I might well have coded Mari-Carmen's
answers as "medically compliant," an instance of a working-
class Spanish-speaker accepting the authority of medicine rather
passively. I might also have coded her husband's intense Pentecostalist presentation as "Hispanic." But once she described the
real risks in her life—a dangerous neighborhood and substan-
dard schools for her children; a husband involved in drugs and
other threats to family stability—I came to believe that Mari-
Carmen had accepted the amniocentesis as a very small part of
a larger design for family stabilization she was actively developing. "Hispanic" values of family and community clearly influenced her ability to welcome both Jesus and genetics into that
strategy. These cultural values, though, are mobilized in the
specific socioeconomic context in which she now lives. There
is no way to disaggregate the class-inflected risks of neighborhood and the illicit networks threatening her family from the
cultural resources and values she used to protect it.

When I interviewed an African-American Wall Street secretary about her decision not to have an amniocentesis at age 37,
she spoke about her husband's reaction to the consent form they
were asked to sign. The form only covered lab procedures for
analyzing the chromosomes extracted through the test; it was
not a permission to perform the test, which is inscribed in different documents. But the lab form, which is written in quite
technical language (and often skimmed or skipped by those
committed to undergoing testing) included a proviso to use dis-
carded amniotic fluid anonymously for experimentation. Reading intensively, the husband was disturbed by this clause, citing
the Tuskegee syphilis experiments and other examples of abusive research conducted on black people as his reason for rejecting the test. Scientific bureaucratese here touched a culturally
and historically sensitive memory of racially abusive medical
domination.

When a well-known, upper middle-class WASP economist heard about this research, she told me her own amniocentesis story: pregnant with a third child at 38, she read extensively in the medical literature, and discovered that the birthrate of live-born children with Down syndrome was 25% lower than the figures quoted for the prenatal detection of this condition. She reasoned that the test was less accurate (that is, that it produced 25% false positives) than the geneticists were claiming, and rejected it on that basis. The difference between the two rates (at midtrimester, via amniocentesis; at birth, among liveborns) is, of course, based on another "fact" which she failed to turn up in her reading: chromosomally atypical fetuses remain vulnerable to miscarriage and stillbirth throughout the pregnancy; late spontaneous abortions of Down fetuses account for the difference in rates. Her "informed consent" to reject the test was based on a strategy I have often observed among white, upper middle-class professionals: they "fight with numbers," testing whether the discourse of genetics actually includes their own particular case and can respond to their sophisticated but idiosyncratic statistical interpretations. They feel comfortable deploying the language of statistics, using this strategy to accept or reject the counselor's expertise. The white economist's rejection was thus based on her cultural values and background no less than that of the African-American secretary.

Attitudes, knowledge, and beliefs about disabling conditions are also highly variable, and they enter into the decisions regarding acceptance and refusal of the test. For example, in two cases of the same diagnosis (the sex chromosome anomaly, Klinefelter syndrome), the same decision to end the pregnancy was made. But in one case, a middle-class professional couple said they "didn't want the pregnancy if he can't have a shot at growing up to be president," while a recently immigrated working-class couple said, "it isn't fair to impose this burden, too, on a child." A young Puerto Rican welfare mother continued her pregnancy after a prenatal diagnosis of Klinefelter. When I interviewed her four years later, during a second amniocentesis for a subsequent pregnancy, she was confident about her growing son's abilities, stressing that Klinefelter syndrome was not a physical disability. "As long as he looks normal, I'll be there for him," she told me. It is important not to romanticize her reactions; initially sent for amniocentesis because she had a sister disabled by spina bifida, she would have aborted for that diagnosis. And a few months ago I learned of a Puerto Rican family dilemma being played out over another diagnosis of a sex chromosome problem, which the father interpreted as a code for homosexuality, despite the genetic counselors' best efforts. When diagnoses involve sex chromosomes, they often index anxieties about the limits of the natural bases of sexuality. A Colombian manicurist, for example, married to a Dominican factory worker, received a fetal diagnosis of Klinefelter. At their counseling session, they did not express much concern about the 10–20% risk of learning disabilities or mental retardation that accompanies this syndrome, and they listened to discussions of gynocomastia (male breast enlargement) and micropenises without intense distress. But the husband asked, "Is this going to make him homosexual? I don't want that." And the wife said, "He won't be able to have children—I wonder if he'll blame us." Both expressed concern about knowing something hidden that the son wouldn't know about himself, at least until he was older.

Culturally specific heritages also enter into how children born with disabilities are assimilated into family life. An African-American welfare-dependent mother of three told me this story about the birth of her son with Down syndrome: She had been planning to put the newborn up for adoption, a decision she had reached shortly before his birth, due to the domestic stress and violence with which she was living. When the baby was born and diagnosed, a white social worker came to see her about placing the child. The mother asked what would become of her baby and was told, "We'll probably find a rural farm family to take him." "Then what?" she queried. "He'll grow up outside, knowing about crops and animals," was the reply. "Then what?" the mother repeated. "Maybe he'll even grow up to work on that farm," the social worker replied. "Sounds like slavery to me," answered the mother, who decided to take her baby home. This imagery and its legacy contrasts strongly the stories of many white mothers who often fantasize peaceful, outdoor, small-scale life as the perfect placement for their children with Down syndrome. The following story was told by a white, Jewish nurse who had a seven-year-old with Down: "I read somewhere that there's a community for retarded people in the mountains, somewhere in Europe. They play music and they run a farm. Kids like this are very loving, they're good with animals, it's like the music of the universe is inside of them. If only the rest of us could listen, maybe they could teach us to hear it better."

The point of all these stories is quite simple: Those culturally specific, historical legacies deeply influence how the offer of an amniocentesis or an abortion for a fetus affected by a genetic disorder is placed in the foreground or background of consciousness. Some risks are more experience-near or experience-far, as anthropologists would describe them (Geertz, 1968), based on the ways in which class and culture shape any particular woman's aspirations for herself and her family, and the resources she has at her disposal when making a medical decision. The resources of class and culture are deeply embedded in any individual woman's particular life history, where they intersect the myriad personal experiences on which her understandings of medicine, maternity, abortion, and disabled children (among many other factors) are shaped. This complex intersection of what is socially structured and what is more individually acquired in any personal biography should alert us against accepting easy stereotypes to explain any particular woman's reproductive decision-making. Yet such stereotypes too frequently emerge when we attempt to generalize about cultural backgrounds. For example, Puerto Ricans, Dominicans, and some other Spanish-speaking groups appear far more concerned about visibly stigmatizing conditions (and more accepting of mental retardation), while white, upper middle-class women and their supporters are more likely to use a medical vocabulary and assume that mental retardation diagnosed in their fetus is cause for abortion.

It would be a mistake, however, to jump too quickly to ethnic-racial explanations of such differences in attitude for several reasons: First, the factors noted above—differential access, the problem of prior knowledge and familiarity with scientific vocabulary and world-view, and the issue of relative trust versus suspicion of their local health care institutions—all affect what women will do. Second, as every counselor knows, individual reproductive and life history are also powerful factors. I spoke recently with a 42-year-old white middle-class woman who was in the throes of making a decision to continue or end a pregnancy after a diagnosis of trisomy 18, a profoundly disabling and usually fatal condition. Her anguish about the possibility of never being able to become pregnant again was clearly central to the decision she was making. And several years ago I interviewed an Italian-American Catholic homemaker, mother of three, who identified with the right-to-life movement, but who had aborted after a prenatal diagnosis of Down. Among the reasons she gave was her strong love for her daughter, whose life she imagined would be taken over by caring for the disabled sibling after her own death. She thus described her abortion as "an act of love."

The Impact of Prenatal Genetic Testing on Women

The impact of prenatal genetic testing should be assessed with women's diversity of perspectives squarely in mind. Otherwise, the design of future research and services will reproduce the inequalities of access, relevance, and power women currently already experience. We need to consider the implications of amniocentesis for the many women and their supporters whose lives it affects: health care providers and pregnant patients; parents of children with disabilities and the larger population whose attitudes, knowledge, and beliefs about disabilities both shape and are shaped by mass media, education, health care, and other social services. Amniocentesis (or any other piece of reproductive technology) intersects a woman's life in relation to all its other problems and possibilities: class, racial, and ethnic markers. Experiences with, and attitudes toward, a range of disabilities all strongly influence a woman's response to the test. We need to insist simultaneously on the collective and individual nature of those orienting features each woman brings to her encounter with prenatal testing. It matters whether one is African-American, Polish- or Irish-Catholic, middle-class or working-class or working-poor. But it also matters whether this is a first or a fourth pregnancy, whether you have experienced difficulties in becoming and staying pregnant, whether you had a cousin with Down or a neighbor who had hemophilia.

There is no simple "feminist" response to the question of whether amniocentesis (or any other piece of reproductive technology) is liberatory or socially controlling because it is always potentially both, depending on the weight various social and individual experiences hold in a particular woman's life. Early feminist writings on amniocentesis suggested it was another "male takeover" of female nature (Corea, 1985; Spallone & Skinberg, 1987). I share a general feminist suspicion of who develops and controls access to new technologies, especially in the realm of reproductive medicine, where women have served as metaphorical handmaidens and material guinea pigs to Western science throughout its history (Jordanova, 1986, 1989). But I am also suspicious of an antitechnological stance, particularly when the majority of women may still be fighting for access to some of the same biomedical technologies over which a minority has raised important criticisms. The intersecting fault lines of class, race, ethnic and religious differences, sexual preference, experiences with disabling conditions, and so forth all must influence our ongoing awareness of a need for both access and complex protections with regard to this, or any other, piece of medical technology.

Clearly, issues of gender and power weave through my current research, but their effects are multiple and never simple. I have certainly seen women pressured into the position of being "agents of quality control on the reproductive production line" by husbands (Rothman, 1986). But I have also seen women using amniocentesis above their male partner's objections. And pro-choice or anti-abortion attitudes may create schisms across gender divides within households and families. We need to locate our understandings of reproductive technologies in relation to the issues on which women might come together—the need for respectful, accessible health care; protection and expansion of reproductive rights in their full complexity. But we also need to confront the issues that potentially divide us: class-based access to differential health care, racial discrimination, and discrimination against adults and children with disabilities.

A second factor in assessing the impact of prenatal genetic

testing on women concerns the sensitivity of health care providers. Genetic counseling is a relatively new health care profession, and 95% of its practitioners are women. There are currently many "women's professions" emerging in health care,
like genetic counseling, in which women speak both the languages of science and of social work, of epidemiology and of
empathy. Counselors are taught to think about "psychosocial"
issues using a neo-Freudian vocabulary. I am suggesting that
there are also social and cultural issues at stake, and these, too,
need to be discussed in the training of genetic counselors. Here,
further research is certainly needed. Recently, Diana Punales-
Morejon and I conducted a preliminary survey of the 15 heads
of genetic counseling training programs in North America, and
of 50 counselors who are particularly experienced in providing
genetic services to minority and underserved populations. Our
data reveal a great deal of ferment in the field over appropriate
education for urban health care careers (Punales-Morejon &
Rapp, 1991; Rapp, 1993a). What, for example, is the role of
language training and familiarity with multicultural attitudes
and aspirations toward pregnancy, testing, abortion, and childhood disability in genetic counselor training programs? We are
convinced that this is a good time to build additional multicultural awareness into a small, but growing, and still-self-
conscious "women's profession."

There is one additional area that should be assessed in thinking about the impact of prenatal genetic testing on women: the
influence of the mass media. While this issue appears to take us
far afield from health care providers and their clients, it is a
critical arena in which awareness, attitudes, and values are constructed. I have been consistently impressed by the role that TV
talk shows, docudramas, science programs, and soap operas
play, especially in the science education of women from non-
privileged backgrounds. After a Phil Donahue show featuring
parent-activists of children with Down syndrome, clinic patients asked much more insightful questions about amniocentesis. The popularity of "Life Goes On" (starring a young adult
with Down syndrome) has raised important issues in both the
genetic services community, and among parents of children
with this condition. A mother of a six-year-old with Down told

me that the single greatest weapon against the stigma her son faced was the inclusion of teenagers with Down in the Mac-Donald's ads. Dorothy Nelkin and Susan Lindee have just completed a survey and analysis of the popular media representations of genes and genetic testing (Lindee & Nelkin, 1994). It is apparent that the density and complexity of coverage of this and related issues is expanding rapidly. A recent *New England Journal of Medicine* article suggests that doctors, too, take their citation cues from stories covered in the *New York Times* (Phillips, Kanter, Bednarczyk, & Tastad, 1991). Science writing and scientific topics have become an integral part of popular culture, for better and for worse, and like all resources in our culture, they are highly stratified and targeted. We need to know more about how stories on genetic testing and its consequences are produced and consumed. I do not intend a naive recommendation that "popular education" alone will enhance our ability to deal with the complex issues of eugenics and reproductive rights that lie at the heart of genetic testing. But surely, we need to imagine (and advocate for) greater public understandings— understandings that take place throughout all strata of our society, and that are removed from the aura of crisis so often accompanying both prenatal diagnosis and the birth of children with disabilities. Scientific literacy is a benefit and a burden affecting all whose lives are touched by reproductive genetic testing. Taking media representations and media access seriously is part of evaluating the impact of reproductive genetic testing, and reproductive technology in general, on the lives of women and their supporters.

ACKNOWLEDGMENTS

Portions of this study have been funded by the National Science Foundation, the National Endowment for the Humanities, a Changing Gender Roles Fellowship from the Rockefeller Foundation, the Institute for Advanced Study (Princeton, NJ), the Spencer Foundation, and a sabbatical semester from the New School for Social Research. I am grateful to them all, and absolve them of any responsibility for the uses I have made of their support. I want to thank the many health professionals who have aided this work because they believed in the necessity of better understanding their patients' experiences. Above all, I am grateful to the many pregnant women, mothers of children with disabilities, and their supporters who shared their amniocentesis stories with me. All of their names have been changed to protect their confidentiality. This article builds on work reported in Rapp, 1994; 1993a; and 1993b. It has benefited immeasurably from the collegial support of Diana Punales-Morejon, for which I am, as ever, grateful.

BIBLIOGRAPHY

COREA, G. (1985). *The mother machine.* New York: Harper & Row.

COWAN, R. S. (1992). Genetic technology and reproductive choice: An ethics for autonomy. In D. J. Kevles & L. Hood (Eds.), *The code: Scientific and social issues in the Human Genome Project* (pp. 244–263). Cambridge, MA: Harvard University Press.

COWAN, R. S. (1993). Aspects of the history of prenatal diagnosis. *Fetal Diagnosis and Therapy, 8*(S1, April), 10–17.

GEERTZ, C. (1968). From the native's points of view. In K. Basso and H. Selby (Eds.), *Meaning in anthropology* (pp. 221–238). Albuquerque: University of New Mexico Press.

HSU, L. (1989, June 10). Portrait of the prenatal diagnosis laboratory: A tenth anniversary report [unpublished lecture delivered at New York University Medical School].

JORDANOVA, L. (1986). *Languages of nature.* Minneapolis: University of Minnesota Press.

JORDANOVA, L. (1989). *Sexual visions.* London: Verso.

LINDEE, S., & Nelkin, D. (1994). *Supergene: DNA in popular culture.* New York: W. H. Freeman.

MCDONOUGH, P. (1990). Congenital disability and medical research: The development of amniocentesis. *Women and Health, 16*(3/4), 137–153.

MEDICAL and Health Research Association, Inc. (1990). *An assessment of unmet needs for genetic services in New York City, 1988: Final report and supplement.* New York: Medical and Health Research Association, Inc., and Department of Health.

PHILLIPS, D., Kanter, E., Bednarczyk, B., & Tastad, P. (1991). Importance of the lay press in the transmission of medical knowledge to the scientific community. *New England Journal of Medicine, 325*(16), 1180–1183.

PUNALES, D., & Rapp, R. (1991). Genetic counselor training and ethnocultural sensitivity [Poster]. Washington, DC: International Congress of Human Genetics.

RAPP, R. (1993a). Amniocentesis in sociocultural perspective. *Journal of Genetic Counseling, 2*(3), 183–196.

RAPP, R. (1993b). Sociocultural differences in the impact of amniocentesis. *Fetal Diagnosis and Therapy, 267,* 1–7.

RAPP, R. (1994, forthcoming). Risky business: Genetic counseling in a shifting world. In J. Schneider & R. Rapp (Eds.), *Articulating hidden histories*. Berkeley: University of California Press.

ROTHMAN, B. K. (1986). *The tentative pregnancy*. New York: Viking.

SPALLONE, P., & Steinberg, D. (Eds.). (1987). *Made to order*. Elmsford, NY: Pergamon.

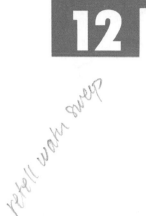

12 Reproductive Genetic Services for Low-Income Women and Women of Color:

Access and Sociocultural Issues

LAURIE NSIAH-JEFFERSON

Implications of Reproductive Technologies

The recent development of new reproductive technologies has dramatically altered the experience of conceiving, carrying to term, and giving birth. At first glance, the new technologies appear to offer women greatly expanded choices regarding whether they conceive, how they conceive, and the health of the child they produce. While reproductive technology may have a positive and desirable impact on some individuals, the implications for society as a whole, however, are mixed.

For example, the very availability of prenatal diagnosis in combination with the availability of abortion may place pressure on parents to use prenatal technologies (Andrews, 1987)—particularly those parents who think they lack the resources to raise a child with special needs. A possible devaluation and stigmatization of people with genetic defects may follow. The availability of prenatal knowledge of genetic "problems" assumes that such conditions can be avoided. The growth of prenatal screening technology, therefore, could foster an environment in which society no longer feels responsible for disabled people.

The ways in which societal questions concerning reproductive issues are framed further complicate matters. Especially troublesome is the assumption that individuals are privately responsible for "solving" genetic problems. Andrews argues that

234

new reproductive technologies focus upon genetic causes while de-emphasizing environmental causes of illness (1987). Rothman criticizes the effect of procedures such as amniocentesis as privatizing a public health problem. She believes that a health care system that stresses prenatal diagnosis and subsequent abortion of "defective" fetuses will place less emphasis on research into the causes and treatment of genetic diseases (1986).

Although the new reproductive technologies affect all women and parents to some degree, the extent of those ramifications will vary according to class position and racial and ethnic identity. Taken from a historical perspective, it is conceivable that in the future poor people might be coerced to abort due to the perceived economic burden on society of having a disabled child. It is also conceivable that in the future poor people might be denied full access to those technologies. As a result, their children would disproportionately represent the population of those with special needs.

To further explore the implications of reproductive genetic technology on low-income women and women of color, the following areas will be discussed: (1) access and barriers to general prenatal care and reproductive genetic services; (2) the availability of reproductive genetic services through public programs and funding; (3) sociocultural issues involved in genetic counseling; and (4) conclusions and recommendations for improving the quality of access to reproductive genetic services.

Access to Prenatal and Reproductive Genetic Services for the Poor: Financial and Systems Barriers

The Uninsured

Many poor women do not utilize prenatal care because they are uninsured. A study by Brown in 1988 showed that of an estimated 9 million women of childbearing age, 1,530,000 (17%) were uninsured altogether, while an additional 5 million were uninsured for prenatal care. Among women of childbearing age, the following statistics were documented for the uninsured women, by demographic status: 23% were unmarried; 22% were 15–19 years old; 27% were 20–24 years old; 21%

were black and 28% were Hispanic; 35% were below the poverty level and 33% had incomes at 100 to 149% of the poverty level; 25% had fewer than 12 years of education; 20% were from the South; and 29% were from the West. Studies point out that privately insured women are more likely to obtain adequate prenatal care, including specialized care, than are those who are uninsured or on Medicaid (Brown, 1988).

Acceptance of Medicaid Patients

Many Medicaid recipients lack access to prenatal care because a large number of obstetricians will not accept Medicaid as a form of payment. In 1983 a national survey of private physicians who provided obstetric care found that 44% did not accept Medicaid. Although states have made efforts to address this issue over the years, the situation has not changed significantly. In large part, the problem is due to the fact that physicians do not receive full reimbursement for their services through Medicaid. Many physicians, however, feel that high-risk Medicaid patients are more apt than non–Medicaid patients to sue their providers (Rosenbaum, Hughes, & Johnson, 1988). According to a 1992 American College of Obstetrics and Gynecology survey, rising malpractice rates have led more than 23% of all responding physicians to reduce their high-risk caseloads. Many physicians have stopped treating high-risk mothers and babies on their premises to avoid legal liability (Rosenbaum et al., 1988).

Waiting Periods in Minority Clinics

The length of the waiting period for obtaining prenatal care in federally funded Maternal and Child Health (MCH) programs greatly influences the feasibility of obtaining prenatal screening. The average waiting period for new patients is about three weeks, but the average length varies from state to state. In 1986, six states had an average waiting period of one week or less, but in 12 states it was four weeks or more. The average waiting period in Vermont was 14 weeks, clearly precluding early entry into prenatal care (AGI, 1987). A long waiting period affects the practicality of utilizing certain prenatal procedures, and this is compounded if low-income women seek prenatal care late in their pregnancies. Women receiving prenatal care late may be rushed through the counseling and screening process; as a result, they may be unable to absorb the information or psychologically prepare for tests, increasing the likelihood of unwise decisions being made.

Long waiting periods for access to prenatal screening particularly affect women who enter prenatal care late in their pregnancies. Compared to white women, a high percentage of black women receive inadequate care or do not have the recommended number of visits (Children's Defense Fund, 1991), decreasing their chances for counseling at an early stage. Women who enter prenatal care late may request screening as far as 20 weeks into their pregnancies which, in many instances, makes it impossible to schedule counseling, undergo the procedure, obtain the results and, if needed, obtain further counseling.

Provision of Services through Public Programs and Funding

Maternal and Child Health Block Grants (which usually include services for children with special needs), community and migrant health centers (AGI, 1987), state-funded regional genetic centers, and funding through Medicaid all provide some level of reproductive genetic services and prenatal care for low-income patients (AGI, 1987). The federal government also funds genetics programs through demonstration projects, through the Bureau of Maternal and Child Health, for Special Programs of Regional and National Significance (NCEMCH, 1991). Some government programs have been contracting with health maintenance organizations (HMOs) to provide services to low- and moderate-income populations. In addition, the federal government provides some services itself. The Public Health Service, for example, is directed to provide voluntary genetic testing, diagnosis, counseling, and treatment of individuals; some members of the armed services and their families can obtain services through CHAMPUS; and some states provide services on a piecemeal basis for categorical problems such as Tay-Sachs disease. Services can also be obtained through Sup-

plemental Social Security Income (Greenstein, 1987). States ensure access to genetic services by acting as direct providers,
paying for services outright in programs that are specifically
directed at genetics, in addition to requiring others to pay for
testing when it is provided by health professionals in the private
sector (Clayton, 1994).

The cost of reproductive genetic screening, however, often
makes it inaccessible to low-income women and their families.
Services for the poor are generally available through the above-
mentioned programs. Most of those programs, though, limit
access to reproductive genetic services and impose eligibility requirements. These limitations shape availability according to
political and organizational biases and agendas underlying social
policy programs and their funding.

Funding through Medicaid

The Medicaid program, Title XIX of the Social Security Act,
is the nation's major vehicle for financing health care for low-
income persons who receive cash assistance under Aid to Families with Dependent Children or Supplemental Social Security
Income. With the introduction of COBRA legislation, a patient
no longer has to be eligible for cash assistance to be eligible for
Medicaid. Medicaid works through a system of reimbursement
to participating private physicians, hospitals, clinics, laboratories, pharmacies, and other health care providers for designated
services. It is administered within broad federal guidelines, but
individual states decide the categories of persons eligible, income eligibility levels, and the services covered. Therefore, the
medical services available to low-income persons vary from
state to state (AGI, 1987).

Limitations on Clinic Visits

Medicaid patients who have medical indications for reproductive genetic testing require a higher than average number of
visits in order to receive the recommended ultrasound, amniocentesis, counseling, or other services. In 1986, however, only
14 states would reimburse for further visits; in addition, in
many of those states the provider must petition for such reimbursement on a case-by-case basis and must have a medical di-

agnosis. For example, in Colorado and North Carolina additional reimbursement is available when a woman has toxemia, cardiac or neurological problems, or a similar condition. In Florida additional reimbursement is available in cases such as preeclampsia (AGI, 1987). In most instances, visits will already have been rendered by the time reimbursement is requested, meaning that the physician takes a financial risk by proceeding. It is conceivable that a physician may indeed refuse to treat a client once the allotted number of visits have been exhausted.

Access to Screening Procedures

There are a variety of reproductive genetic tests available. For the purposes of this discussion, I will outline a few techniques: Amniocentesis involves inserting a needle through the abdomen of a pregnant woman into the uterus to remove a small amount of amniotic fluid that is tested to determine fetal abnormalities. Ultrasound screening determines fetal position and age and may identify certain fetal abnormalities. Alpha-fetoprotein (AFP) tests are performed to detect abnormalities from a blood sample. Chorionic villi sampling (CVS) is an early diagnostic test that removes from the uterus a piece of chorion, the outer tissue of the sac surrounding the embryo. The chorionic tissue is analyzed to determine the genetic makeup of the fetus. This procedure can test for most of the same chromosomal, metabolic, and other genetic disorders as amniocentesis, but it cannot identify the presence of neural tube defects (Blatt, 1988).

The majority of states provide Medicaid reimbursement for amniocentesis, ultrasound, and AFP. As a general rule, all the procedures required for these particular screening techniques are funded. Connecticut and Kansas provide only partial coverage of amniocentesis, reimbursing the physician fee for the procedure, but failing to reimburse laboratory fees for examining the amniotic fluids (AGI, 1987). In a 50-state analysis of Medicaid reimbursement for medical genetics, it was found that in six states determination for reimbursement for CVS procedures was based on individual consideration on a per-test basis by medical review (Greenstein, 1987).[1] Prenatal testing procedures tend to be expensive. For example, estimates of the costs of amniocentesis (including ultrasound) range from $600 to $2,000 depending upon the institution and the condition for which the testing is being done. However, the mean reimbursement for amniocentesis by Medicaid is significantly less, often not even covering one-half of the cost of the procedure. The low reimbursement rates for these procedures from the Medicaid program reduce the number of physicians willing to provide particular prenatal screening services to low-income women.

Even if low-income women can find private physicians willing to accept Medicaid, they are often faced with qualifying restrictions that act as barriers to obtaining quality prenatal screening service. Some states stipulate restrictions, often based on prior authorization by a physician, the age of the woman, the type of medical complication, or the number of tests previously completed. For example, a low-income woman can obtain ultrasound screening via Medicaid funding in all states except California. However, in New Hampshire she is subject to prior authorization, and in three states (Georgia, Minnesota, and Texas) she is subject to restrictions by age and by particular medical complication, and reimbursed only in those cases in which the procedure is defined as "medically necessary." Other states leave the definition of medical necessity to the discretion of the physician. The variability in definition means that some low-income women may not be able to obtain a particular screening technique in the areas in which they live, despite the fact that the procedure is funded in their state and that they qualify for it in neighboring states.

In Greenstein's 50-state study, between four and six states (depending on the type of counseling provided), did not cover genetic counseling costs, and between three and five provided reimbursement based on individual consideration by medical review (1987). This implies that a woman may have access to one procedure, but not to the counseling that may be necessary to accompany the test. Genetic procedures and results from laboratory tests are only valuable when preceded or accompanied by genetic counseling.[2] The counseling helps couples interpret and think through the results of the test—a difficult and sensitive task.

It should also be noted that in order for genetic counseling to be reimbursed it must be carried out by a physician or a geneticist with a Ph.D. In many instances, these individuals are too overwhelmed with other medical duties to be able to adequately provide counseling services. Many physicians have a genetics counselor, who is part of their practice, provide this care in order that the service be reimbursed. However, recent studies show that the average Medicaid reimbursement for counseling was approximately only one-third of the amount private insurers would reimburse for the same service (Greenstein, 1987).

The lower rate of Medicaid reimbursement and the restrictions on the provision of services contribute to creating a two-tiered medical system that influences access and quality of care for low-income women. Although some restrictions may be medically appropriate (such as considering the age of women) and others may protect poor women and women of color from unwarranted overuse of prenatal screening procedures, overall the restrictions do not allow equal access to high-quality health services. Even in places where prenatal screening is available in terms of geographic location, poor women have less control over the quality of care they receive because only some physicians and clinics choose to participate. Thus, the ability of Medicaid patients to obtain prenatal screening is markedly different from that of middle-class women.

Funding through MCH Programs and Community and Migrant Health Centers

The Maternal and Child Health program has very broad goals, including the promotion of maternal and child health through the provision of basic prenatal care and specialized care to children with disabling conditions. When Congress enacted the MCH Block Grant in 1981, prenatal care and genetic services were two of the programs covered; therefore, reproductive genetic services can be provided from MCH Block Grant funding through maternal and child health and genetic services programs. The income eligibility levels for free or subsidized care vary considerably from state to state, ranging from incomes at 100 to 250% of the poverty level. Three states have no income restrictions whatsoever (AGI, 1987).

Community health centers (CHCs) and migrant health centers (MHCs) provide services to underserved, disadvantaged populations. Several hundred agencies in urban and rural areas

of 49 states receive federal funds for reproductive genetic services (NCPCI, 1986). Two-thirds of the clients belong to minority groups and six out of ten have incomes below the federal
poverty level. An additional 25% have incomes between 100
and 200% of the federal poverty level. Perinatal care services are
included in the authorizing legislation that defines the primary
care services that must be provided by CHCs and MHCs. Physician, laboratory, and other services relevant to maternity care
must also be provided.[3]

While CHCs generally provide a broad range of services including education, counseling, and social services, the medical
care related to pregnancy appears to be fairly basic. Thirty-four
percent of those agencies that do provide prenatal care do not
serve high-risk patients on-site. Twenty-two percent of the
CHCs and MHCs that only service low-risk patients on-site
offer paid referrals for high-risk patients (AGI, 1987).

An examination of the funding of prenatal screening techniques through MCH programs and CHC and MHC services
reveals two patterns that hamper equal access for low-income
women. First, prenatal screening procedures are generally
available in fewer states through MCH programs, CHCs, and
MHCs than the number of states that provide specific services
through Medicaid funding. For instance, only 48% of CHCs
and MHCs and 80% of the country's MCH programs fund or
provide ultrasound as compared to the 96% of states that fund
the procedure through Medicaid (although as mentioned above,
two states only provide partial coverage). The pattern is similar
for coverage for amniocentesis and other related procedures
(AGI, 1987).

The second pattern relates to the difference in the services
offered through the MCH programs and the CHCs and MHCs.
Overall, fewer states fund prenatal screening techniques
through CHCs and MHCs than through MCH programs. For
example, 72% of the states provide or pay for amniocentesis in
MCH programs, while only 48% of the states provide or pay
for this procedure in CHCs or MHCs (AGI, 1987). Furthermore, some clients are asked to pay a small fee.

It is important to note that women who have access to Medicaid but receive their services through these clinics also face

limited coverage, unless referred to a facility that accepts Medicaid. Such women should be made aware of the fact that if they are referred elsewhere additional procedures may be covered (although many women with Medicaid only have access to clinic services).

Overall it is clear that low-income women or women of color who use these clinics have more restricted access to prenatal screening techniques than women who utilize Medicaid services, and far more restricted access than women who have other forms of third-party coverage.

Special Programs for Pregnant Women

Some states have special maternity programs for women who are eligible for Medicaid and/or public assistance. There are also programs available for women who have low incomes, but incomes that are above the eligibility requirements for Medicaid. The first type of program has special provisions to determine eligibility in a short period of time and to provide a more comprehensive package of services for pregnant women. Most of these programs provide presumptive eligibility for women, allowing them to receive prenatal care services while actual eligibility for Medicaid is determined (Brown, 1988). Such programs allow women to enter prenatal care earlier in their pregnancies than would be the case if they applied for Medicaid without the benefit of this special program, and they also allow women to be evaluated for high-risk conditions including those that would require prenatal screening and testing. However, although these programs do offer the services of a nutritionist, health educator, case manager, and other specialists, most do not provide the services of a genetics assistant or genetics education on-site. Such provision could greatly increase referral and follow-up for potential genetic problems that affect some low-income populations—problems indicated by factors such as hemoglobin variants, being older than 35, HIV-positive status, and teratogen exposure from working in a dangerous environment, or substance abuse. Nevertheless, these programs do provide much-needed early prenatal care and screening services.

The second type of special program provides services to

women whose incomes are too high for Medicaid but too low to comfortably afford private insurance. One such program is the Healthy Start Program in Massachusetts. In 1985 the program accommodated women who were not currently enrolled in Medicaid, had no private insurance, and had a family income at or below 200% (originally 185%) of the federal poverty level. Healthy Start also underwrote the initial cost of the women's eligibility for Medicaid. All necessary medical care to maintain health during pregnancy is covered, including prenatal screenings, plus one pediatric visit. Providers are reimbursed at Medicaid rates for physicians at CHCs and at non-Medicaid public assistance rates for hospitals (Brown, 1988). It is up to the individual states to determine what types of procedures will be covered by such programs. In most cases, to control program costs (as with all public programs), there are some financial constraints and limitations put on the services provided to clients. Program evaluators have shown that this initiative has increased the number of low-income women able to access prenatal care (Brown, 1988) and should consequently have increased the number of women accessing reproductive genetic services at some level.

Reproductive Genetics Offered through HMOs

Some people with low incomes receive their care through HMOs, either through employment-based services or through state case management. For instance, in recent years an increasing number of states have begun to contract on a prepaid basis with providers of comprehensive health services, such as HMOs. Under these plans a local health care provider agrees to provide all or most of the needed health services to a patient for a fixed fee paid monthly or annually in advance. This kind of plan, called capitation, enables states to control costs by shifting the financial risk associated with paying for unexpected major medical problems from the state to the local provider.

The provision of care through HMOs is not, however, well matched to the realities of reproductive genetics. Because HMO policy discourages using specialists, HMO providers may not refer patients as often as they should for services or procedures (Pyeritz, 1990; Kenney, Torres, Dittes, & Mocias, 1986). In addition, HMOs normally contract with one laboratory. If the medical center to which a patient is referred for testing uses a different laboratory than the one contracted by the HMO, laboratory procedures may not be reimbursed. This situation may force the medical center to absorb the cost for low- or moderate-income patients.

Although HMOs have achieved considerable presence in a short time, with a few exceptions, they have not resolved how to deliver genetic services. At the present time, few HMOs believe they are large enough to support a full-time geneticist and genetics laboratory. Referrals outside the plan are expensive and are often viewed as a drain on potential profits (Pyeritz, 1990). Nevertheless, HMOs are beginning to address access to genetic services. Blake conducted a statewide assessment of financial access to genetic services in New York State and found that some form of coverage was provided for genetic services. Claims for genetic services in New York are paid if ordered by a patient's physician, the patient being referred if she has a history of miscarriage, has previously given birth to a child with a genetic disorder, or is in a high-risk group. In addition, it was found that genetic services were provided both by in-house HMO group members and by referrals to outside consultants or genetic service centers (Blake, 1987). The number and type of services referred to outside providers varied with each HMO. Eleven of the 17 HMOs surveyed indicated that referrals were sometimes made to non-HMO providers currently recognized as part of the statewide genetic services program (Blake, 1987). Although this is the case in New York State, additional research needs to be conducted on the role of HMOs in the provision of genetic services throughout the country.

Whether services are provided through an HMO or through other programs, the costs of providing care to low-income or culturally different populations are relatively higher than are the costs of providing services to the general population, and reimbursements are proportionately less. For instance, reimbursement is rare for nonphysician services that may be involved in the care of low-income or foreign-born patients, such as interpreters, additional social service referrals, nursing services, or genetics counselors or assistants (March of Dimes, 1990).

Access to Abortion

Abortion following prenatal diagnosis is fully available through Medicaid in just 13 states. Ten states fund abortion through Medicaid only in instances in which the woman's life is endangered, while other states impose varying restrictions, such as providing funding only when the pregnancy is a result of a rape or incest (Daley & Benson-Gold, 1993). Federal employees, recipients of services from the Indian Health Services (IHS), and federal inmates are also subject to such restrictions. For example, during fiscal year 1987, the Bureau of Prisons paid for an abortion only when the life of the mother would have been endangered if the fetus were carried to term or if the pregnancy was a result of rape. Most of these limitations do not allow a woman who has a "defective" fetus to have an abortion with public funding. For federal inmates, their sole source of medical care is through the prison, and for Native Americans who are geographically isolated from towns and cities, the IHS may in reality be their only source of health care. For those populations, then, access to abortion is very limited.

In instances where a woman chooses to terminate her pregnancy after an undesirable test result, the financial costs may be prohibitive—particularly in the case of a late-term abortion, which usually costs about $900. Poor women, thus, have very few options unless the abortions are performed at low or no cost. Public hospitals are a major source of health care for the poor, yet only 17% of all public hospitals report having performed abortions in 1985 (Henshaw, Forrest, & VanVort, 1987). Poor women also have limited access to facilities that provide abortions after the first trimester. Because so few providers perform late-term abortions, locating a facility, scheduling the procedure, and arranging travel can all impose serious burdens (Boston Women's Health Book Collective, 1986).

Professional and Public Education and Referral Systems

Because reproductive genetics is a relatively new and constantly changing field, public and medical providers require current, up-to-date information on procedures and services. Primary health care providers, too, need to have a basic knowledge of the various genetic diseases, the related tests, and their implications. They need to know how to conduct the prescreening in order to identify patients at potential risk, and they need to be able to convey this information to low-income clients in a comprehensive manner in order to educate them on their full range of options (Paul & Kavanaugh, 1990). Ways in which to effectively educate the public should be further explored.

Referral systems should also be examined to ensure an effective system that takes into consideration the special needs of low-income patients. As is the case with other medical services, programs serving low-income patients may need increased mechanisms to facilitate follow-up, including telephone follow-up and pre-referral services (Paul & Kavanaugh, 1990). An active relationship between genetic services units and community clinics can involve those clinics in providing ongoing education about the referral process.

Geographic Access

In many states, genetic testing and counseling centers are located at major medical centers; depending on the state, there may be one or several sites. Most centers utilize a sliding-fee scale to assist families who have few resources for payment. In most of these programs, all services offered to more affluent patients are available to low-income clients, regardless of their ability to pay.

Some low-income women, however, may not be able to utilize services available in their state because the prenatal services are unevenly distributed geographically and are targeted to urban women. Research shows that women are more likely to use amniocentesis if they live in metropolitan rather than rural areas and if they have higher education levels (AGI, 1987). These findings hold regardless of race. It has also been found that women living in the South are less likely to have an amniocentesis. The subgroup utilizing the highest proportion of amniocentesis services tend to be white women older than 35 residing in areas other than the South (AGI, 1987). These findings seem to indicate that black women residing in the rural South may have especially limited access to reproductive genetic services.

Some studies, in addition, show that women who live in rural areas and are less educated are more likely to be subjected to prenatal screening using x-rays (AGI, 1987). According to a 1987 study, x-ray screening was performed on some women despite the fact that exposure to x-rays during pregnancy poses an unnecessary, albeit small, risk to the fetus, and that "it has been estimated that one-third of [the] individuals that had x-rays could have had an ultrasound for the same purposes (determining fetal position, fetal age, and multiple pregnancy)" (AGI, 1987). The higher rate of x-ray screening for rural women and for less educated women may be due to several factors: ultrasound technology and personnel may not always be available, clients may be less informed about the danger of x-rays to fetal health, or physicians may have less regard for their clients' health. Regardless of the cause, the more frequent use of x-ray screening may produce negative consequences for certain populations (AGI, 1987).

Other prohibitive factors related to geographic access include parking costs, travel time, time taken off from work, and babysitting fees. Many people do not own cars or cannot afford public transportation (Paul & Kavanaugh, 1990); thus, low-income people who live in suburban and rural populations may be hampered in their access to genetic services and so may use them less. In order to improve the availability of genetic services to geographically isolated populations, it is necessary to establish satellite clinics that utilize local resources, to demand adequate financial support for regional medical genetic centers to provide necessary transportation, and to utilize local resources to develop self-help strategies to address unmet needs.

Sociocultural Barriers and Diversity Issues

The goal of genetic counseling is to educate people about possible etiology, prognosis, management, recurrence, risks, options, and resources relating to genetic diseases (Vargas & Wilkerson, 1987). As with any decision-making process, the meanings attached to whatever is being communicated—in this case the results of the screening and the options available— depend upon the individuals involved and their sociocultural environments (Sue, 1981). When the topics being discussed are as emotionally charged and controversial as issues of reproduction and possible abortion, the individual's core values, while too often unexamined or taken for granted, are likely to be tapped.

Among clients, genetic providers, and counselors, a great diversity is created through the multitude of differences in income level, language, culture, religion, and philosophy (Paul & Kavanaugh, 1990). While such variance in our culture is often a source of enrichment, the differences can also create impediments not easily overcome. There are the overt barriers of communication problems caused by language differences between Hispanics, Asians, and other immigrants, and English-speaking Americans. Less overt, however, are the ethnocultural differences, which are perhaps the greatest barrier to receiving care. Basic philosophies, life experiences, values, and histories vary. The emotions and desires of people may be similar from culture to culture, but their expression is often quite different. An inability to interpret nonverbal language or to understand the social pressures or gender roles in the context of another culture may blind caregivers to the psychosocial needs of their clients (Paul & Kavanaugh, 1990).

In addition, when the counselor and the client hold different class, racial, or ethnic positions in society, the interaction is likely to highlight differences in power and even attempts at social control. Low-income women and women of color, coming from communities whose worldviews often differ from the worldviews of the dominant culture and the medical profession, may experience a greater disjunction between their views and the views of the counselors than may white middle-class women. Luker, for example, documents the impact of different class-based worldviews on reproductive issues in her study of activists for and against abortion rights (1984). Hall and Ferree discuss the different structures of abortion attitudes by race (1986).

The new prenatal technologies frame the entire issue of reproduction for all women in terms of the dominant worldview. These technologies embody a definition of a reproductive problem that focuses on the fetus almost to the exclusion of the mother. Both Rothman and Petchevsky graphically depict the way ultrasound procedures foster the definition of the mother as a "habitat" for the fetus, which becomes a "man-in-space" entity falsely assumed to be capable of independent existence (Petchevsky, 1987; Rothman, 1986). The "eclipsing of the pregnant woman's part in childbearing" is evident in the language used to name the new technologies. The phrase "test-tube baby" ignores the nurturing womb; the term "artificial insemination" disguises the "normal" process of conception, pregnancy, and birth once sperm are present; and "surrogacy" discredits the act of pregnancy as part of mothering (Petchevsky, 1987).

But another aspect of the dominant worldview is the historical association between eugenics and most social policy programs addressing the reproductive activities of poor women and women of color. Davis and Gordon both document how the contraceptive movement shifted from birth control to population control for state purposes in the nineteenth century (Gordon, 1977; Davis, 1983). Initially advocated by progressive thinkers, the birth control movement was an attempt to provide women with more reproductive choices. However, by the 1930s the "birth control movement was increasingly absorbed into programs aimed not at self-determination but at social control by the elite" (Gordon, 1977). Policies were promoted to maintain the dominance of the native-born white population while restricting the reproductive activities of other segments such as immigrants, blacks, and Native Americans. Davis points out the political tone of the birth control movement when she notes the class-bias and racism that crept into the movement early on. More and more, it was assumed that poor women, black and immigrant alike, have a "moral obligation to restrict the size of their families." What was demanded as a "right" for the privileged came to be interpreted as a "duty" for the poor (Davis, 1983).

This "duty" of the poor to have fewer children who might need welfare or other governmental services has become an underlying theme of many federally funded programs. One of the most blatant expressions of the population control directive is the involuntary sterilization of women of color. Dreifus documents how medical residents developed their surgical skills by performing tubal ligations on Hispanic women who were un-informed or misinformed of the operation they were undergo-ing (1977). Davis describes several cases in which black teen-agers were sterilized through various governmental agencies including publicly funded birth control clinics (1983). Other studies have indicated high sterilization rates for Native Ameri-can and Puerto Rican women.

Given the increasing feasibility of "selecting good genes," those who are concerned about the new reproductive technolo-gies should also be concerned that we may be entering a new eugenic era (Bowman, 1977). As was the case in the 1920s, an enthusiasm for using genetic makeup to make judgments about social worth has surfaced. Decisions on who has access to the new technologies will continue to be influenced by age and race; and subtle (and not so subtle) pressures will continue to be put on women who are being counseled, according to their socio-economic status.

The use of reproductive technologies is often perceived by poor women and women of color within this tradition of eu-genics and population control. The meanings and values asso-ciated with abortion and having children are often played out between a white, educated genetics counselor and a low-income black or Hispanic client against a historical background of dis-trust, control, and unequal power.

Within this historical context, three dimensions of conflict in worldview are likely to occur for low-income and minority women. First, in many cultures people see themselves as having little control over their fate, feeling as though they should not interfere with the will of God. For example, many Southeast Asians believe that amniocentesis interferes with the natural se-lection of the population, which is considered sacred (Asian Health Project, 1986). Devout Roman Catholics often view dis-ability as God's will. Instead of assuming that all cultures share the same attitudes, it is important to recognize cultural diver-sity, even within the seeming unity of, say, the predominantly Catholic Latino culture (Almquist, 1984). Given the uniqueness of their historical treatments by governmentally funded health services, it is likely that Cuban, Chicano, and Puerto Rican women have different attitudes toward reproductive technology.

Second, culture will affect ideas about how to interact with authority figures and who should be included in the decision-making process within the family structure. Harwood found that some Puerto Rican patients are unwilling to show that they did not understand or agree with an authority figure such as a physician (1981). The medical model assumes that the individual patient is the paramount decision maker for testing and treatment. But for many women of color, other family members—even extended family members—may be of prime significance in the decision-making process (Farfel & Holtzman, 1984).

Third, as discussed in Rayna Rapp's chapter in this book, different individuals and cultural groups have varying perceptions of the levels of disability they can cope with and what it might be like to live with a disability (Rapp, 1994, 1987). These and other dimensions of the worldview will heavily influence the dynamics of the counseling process.

In order to help alleviate potential cultural misunderstandings, some valuable community resources can be drawn upon. For instance, in terms of language problems, the training and employment of capable and sensitive interpreters is crucial; the use of mere translators is not sufficient. Indeed, some languages used in the United States today do not even have a genetics vocabulary (Paul & Kavanaugh, 1990). Bilingual care is the most desirable, and efforts should be made to train minority workers in professional capacities. In addition, an understanding of more than the community's most basic value system is essential. It would do health professionals well to learn about their community's orthodoxy and interpretation without stereotyping. The local clergy can be useful sources in this respect. While at times being unaware or even suspicious of genetic care providers, their knowledge is useful; and they can themselves benefit from an opportunity to learn about genetics, thereby being able to counsel and comfort more effectively (Paul & Kavanaugh, 1990).

Informed Consent

The legal principle that competent adult patients should have autonomy over their bodies is firmly grounded in case law and state statutes (Andrews, 1987). Patient decision-making is protected under the doctrine of informed consent, which requires that a patient's authorization for the diagnostic or treatment option be intentional, substantially noncontrolled, and based on substantial understanding (Faden & Beauchamp, 1986). Informed consent is impaired when clients are not given information (Farfel & Holtzman, 1984) or when the information given is unintelligible or is interpreted through different cultural filters.

Rapp describes how cultural factors can hamper informed consent on at least three levels (Rapp, 1994, 1987). First, certain medical information may not be salient within the sociocultural context of low-income clients. Second, some low-income clients cannot understand the medical terminology being used to interpret the medical information being given. Third, the client may prioritize the medical problems differently from the physician or genetics counselor. Again, given the great impact that decisions relating to informed consent can have on a woman's life, the various sociocultural issues need to be specifically addressed to this question.

Confidentiality

Confidentiality in the prenatal screening process is an extremely important issue for women of color who, historically, have experienced adverse consequences when intimate information has been revealed to third parties. Prenatal screening increases the amount and type of information included in medical files which, if revealed, could harm the patient's reputation, increase family conflict, or restrict education or employment opportunities (Winslade, 1982). Negative consequences have been documented for sickle-cell trait carriers when information was made available to third parties: employers refused to hire, promote, or even retain identified workers, and insurance companies either refused health and life insurance coverage or inflated the cost of coverage despite the fact that the sickle-cell trait has not been linked to shortened life spans (Hubbard & Henifin, 1984).

People with low incomes tend to be at higher risk of having their confidentiality rights abused. Many belonging to the low-income population, such as unwed mothers, adolescent parents, and people at risk of contracting AIDS, have been categorized as being socially "deviant." The disclosure of personal information about them, because they have not adhered to society's moral codes, can have an especially negative impact on their lives. Unwed adolescent women, for example, may fear that the knowledge of their sexual activity or pregnancy will be revealed to their parents, while unwed male partners may fear that their identity will be revealed to public officials pursuing child support payments (Bowman, 1977). A woman may herself avoid prenatal care if she fears that she will be required to involve her male partner in genetic screening.

Conclusions and Recommendations

Although most prenatal screening techniques may be partially funded and available, poor women do not have equal access to them. To provide all women with the option of using reproductive genetic techniques and to make it a personal choice to utilize these techniques, it is imperative that all families have financial, geographic, and social access to prenatal diagnostic procedures.

Funding is a key, but not the only ingredient in this recommendation; information about the availability and purpose of these technologies should be effectively communicated to the public, and the existing qualifying restrictions should be evaluated and removed or modified should they be found to function as barriers to access. Funding should extend to more than only the poorest women who qualify for Medicaid. As has already been done in many states, the state and community should be funders of last resort for the poor who are ineligible for Medicaid or private insurance.

In genetic counseling involving poor women and women of color, it is important that differing worldviews and other potential barriers be considered by health care providers. One solution is that informed consent forms be required and written in simple understandable terms, in languages appropriate to the communities in which they are distributed. In addition, test results, particularly those involving sensitive areas, should be kept confidential and not as part of the patient's medical record. Legal provisions guaranteeing confidentiality should be strengthened.

Furthermore, the negative influence of cultural factors in the counseling process should be addressed specifically. First, minority genetics counselors should be recruited: Black, Latino, and Asian health professionals, including social workers, physicians, counselors, nurses, and auxiliary health workers, should be encouraged to pursue some level of training in genetic counseling to increase the availability of counselors who are familiar with the culture, religion, and language of the community being served and who may understand or share that community's attitudes toward death, disease, disability, and abortion. This approach has been successfully implemented in a number of genetics projects throughout the country.

Second, graduate genetic counseling curricula should include courses on counseling culturally diverse populations, and graduates of past programs should be informed of the availability of continuing education in this area. Where such courses are not available, they should be instituted, and licensing agencies should emphasize the need for such courses. Representatives of the minority groups to be served should be involved in the design, development, and operation of graduate education as well as in the actual medical provision of services.

Instead of merely identifying certain medical or utilization-related characteristics of population groups and service providers, it is important to identify clearly the barriers and gaps in services, and to analyze nationwide what constitute successful strategies. Once this information is gathered it is imperative that it is disseminated to service providers, advocacy groups, and state and local professional and government services to be reviewed and utilized for policy and program development. Additionally, if we are ever going to identify the underserved and document where they live and how well programs designed to serve them are succeeding, we will have to build a minimal base of data, working with the regional and state data coordinators to do special data collection and analysis.

The basic purpose of reproductive genetic technologies ought to be to provide a woman with as much relevant information as possible so that she can make an informed and responsible decision. Between the theory and the actual practice of this ideal, however, there exists an enormous gap. Only by questioning our faith in technological progress, by illuminating the larger framework of medical care and reproduction, can the needs of low-income women and women of color be met. Placing their needs and experiences at the center of any analysis of reproductive technologies brings to the light the operation of ideological as well as structural factors that act as impediments to effective health care delivery. So much emphasis currently lies on the furthering of high technology when low-income women need better public health service in general and basic prenatal care in particular, including equal access to available technologies.

If we begin from the perspective of low-income women and women of color, we see that reproductive technology is just one small piece of a health care system that is neither structurally nor ideologically prepared to meet women's needs. Changing this will require more than creating access to any particular technology or developing new technology. Even the most useful technology is only a means, not an end in itself. The social, economic, medical, and legal context in which women's reproductive health concerns are addressed affects all women, and the perspective of low-income women and women of color may help us to recognize this essential truth.

NOTES

1. Information from Greenstein's 1987 study and from the Alan Guttmacher Institute has not been updated because no more recent studies are known that are of a similar or as comprehensive a nature.
2. Greenstein (1987) describes seven levels of genetic counseling, including initial extended, initial intermediate, initial brief, follow-up extended, follow-up intermediate, follow-up brief, and pre-amniocentesis.
3. Sections 330(b)(2)(A), 329(a)(7)(A), 330(b)(3), and 329(a)(6), PHSA.

BIBLIOGRAPHY

ALAN Guttmacher Institute. (1987). *The financing of maternity care in the United States*. New York: Alan Guttmacher Institute.

ALMQUIST, E. (1984). *Race and ethnicity in the lives of minority women.* In J. Freeman (Ed.), *Women: A feminist perspective* (pp. 423–453). Palo Alto, CA: Mayfield Press.

ANDREWS, L. (1987). *Medical genetics: A legal frontier.* Chicago: American Bar Association.

ASIAN Health Project. (1986). *Asian pacific health news.* Los Angeles: Asian Health Project.

BLAKE, T. (1987). Through the looking glass: A statewide assessment of financial access to genetic services. In R. M. Greenstein, G. B. Gardiner, & D. L. Young, (Eds.), *The challenge to provide genetic services* [Conference proceedings]. Hartford, CT: University of Connecticut School of Medicine.

BLATT, R. (1988). *Prenatal tests.* New York: Vintage.

BOSTON Women's Health Book Collective. (1986). *The new our bodies, our selves.* Boston: Boston Women's Health Book Collective.

BOWMAN, J. E. (1977). Is a national program to prevent sickle cell anemia possible? *American Journal of Pediatric Hematology/Oncology, 5*(4), 367–377.

BROWN, S. (1988). *Prenatal care: Reaching mothers, reaching infants.* Washington, DC: Washington National Academy Press.

CHILDREN's Defense Fund. (1991). *The health of America's children.* Washington, DC: Children's Defense Fund.

CLAYTON, E. W. (1994). What the law says about reproductive genetic testing and what it doesn't. In K. H. Rothenberg & E. J. Thomson (Eds.), *Women and prenatal testing: Facing the challenges of genetic technology.* Columbus, OH: Ohio State University Press.

DALEY, D., & Benson-Gold, R. (1993). Public funding for contraception, sterilization, and abortion services, fiscal year 1992. *Family Planning Prospectus, 25*(6).

DAVIS, A. (1983). *Women, race, and class.* New York: Random House.

DREIFUS, C. (1977). Sterilizing the poor. In C. Dreifus (Ed.), *Seizing our bodies: The politics of women's health* (pp. 109–121). New York: Random House.

FADEN, R., & Beauchamp, T., with King, N. (1986). *A history and theory of informed consent.* New York: Oxford University Press.

FARFEL, M., & Holtzman, N. (1984). Education, consent and counseling in sickle cell screening programs: Report of a survey. *American Journal of Public Health, 74,* 373–375.

GORDON, L. (1977). *Woman's body, woman's right.* Hammondsworth, England: Penguin.

GREENSTEIN, R. M. (1987). Assessment of reimbursement for genetics diseases. In R. M. Greenstein, G. B. Gardiner, & D. L. Young, (Eds.), *The challenge to provide genetics services: Reimbursement for medical genetic services* [Conference proceedings]. Hartford, CT: University of Connecticut.

HALL, E. T., & Ferree, M. M. (1986). Race differences in abortion attitudes. *Public Opinions, 50,* 193–207.

HARWOOD, A. (1981). *Ethnicity and medical care.* Cambridge, MA: Harvard University Press.

HENSHAW, F., Forrest, J., & VanVort, J. (1987). Abortion services in the United States, 1984 and 1985. *Family Planning Perspectives, 19,* 68.

HUBBARD, R., & Henifin, M. S. (1984). Genetic screening of prospective parents and of workers. In J. M. Humber & R. Almedar (Eds.), *Biomedical ethics reviews* (pp. 92–100). Clifton, NJ: Humana Press.

KENNEY, A., Torres, A., Dittes, N., & Mocias, J. (1986). Medicaid expenditures for maternity and newborn care in America. *Family Planning Perspectives, 18,* 155.

LUKER, K. (1984). *Abortions and the politics of motherhood.* Berkeley: University of California Press.

MARCH of Dimes/Birth Defects Foundation. (1990). In N. Paul & L. Kavanaugh (Eds.), *Recommendations from the National Symposium on Genetic Services for Underserved Populations* (pp. 245–248). Original Article Series, Vol. 26, No. 2. Washington, DC: National Center for Education in Maternal and Child Health.

NATIONAL Center for Education in Maternal & Child Health. (1991). *Maternal & child health bureau: Genetics services abstract of active projects.* Washington, DC: National Center for Education in Maternal and Child Health.

NATIONAL Clearinghouse for Primary Care Information. (1986, Fall). *Community health centers: A quality system for the changing health care market* [Pamphlet]. McLean, VA: National Clearinghouse for Primary Care Information.

PAUL, N., & Kavanaugh, L. (Eds.). (1990). *Recommendations from the National Symposium on Genetic Services For Underserved Populations.* Original Article Series, Vol. 26, No. 2. Washington, DC: National Center for Education in Maternal and Child Health.

PETCHEVSKY, R. (1987). Foetal images: The power of visual culture in the politics of abortion. In *Reproductive technologies: Gender, motherhood, and medicine* (pp. 57–80). Minneapolis: University of Minnesota Press.

PYERITZ, R. E. (1990). Common themes under different types of insurance. In N. Paul & L. Kavanaugh (Eds.), *Recommendations from the Symposium on Genetic Services for Underserved Populations.* Washington, DC: National Center for Education in Maternal and Child Health.

RAPP, R. (1987). *Moral pioneer: Women, men, and fetuses on the frontier of reproductive technologies* [Unpublished lecture] (pp. 12–13). Storrs, CT: University of Connecticut.

RAPP, R. (1994). Women's responses to prenatal diagnosis: A sociocultural perspective on diversity. In K. H. Rothenberg & E. J. Thomson (Eds.), *Women and prenatal testing: Facing the challenges of genetic testing.* Columbus, OH: Ohio State University Press.

ROTHMAN, B. K. (1986). *The tentative pregnancy.* New York: Viking.

ROSENBAUM, S., Hughes, D. C., & Johnson, K. (1988). Maternal and child health services for the medically indigent. *Medical Care, 26*(4).

SUE, D. (1981). *Counseling the culturally different: Theory and practice.* New York: Wiley Press.

VARGAS, A., & Wilkerson, L. (1987). Defining our cultures and bridging the gap. In P. N. Maygarit, & B. Biesher (Eds.), *Strategies in genetics counseling: Religious, cultural, and ethnic influences on the counseling process* (pp. 167–187). Original Articles Series, Vol. 23, No. 6. New York: March of Dimes Birth Defects Foundation.

WINSLADE, W. J. (1982). Confidentiality of medical records: An overview of concepts and legal practices. *Journal of Legal Medicine, 3*, 497–533.

13 The Tentative Pregnancy:

Then and Now

BARBARA KATZ ROTHMAN

There is a certain kind of grim satisfaction in having one's prophecies fulfilled, one's concerns justified. I experienced that to a certain extent through the writing of *The Tentative Pregnancy* (1986) as hypotheses became theses, and I have felt it even more so as the years have gone by. To give a brief background of my project, the following questions and answers highlight the major issues discussed in the book:

What are the constraints on the choice to use or not to use prenatal diagnosis and selective abortion in a pregnancy medically defined as "at risk"? The constraints are probably just as one would expect: familial pressure, husband pressure, medical pressure, economic pressure. Some women experience the pressures all from one direction, while some women find themselves at the center of pressures working in powerful opposition to each other (husbands saying one thing, doctors another). Some women are better positioned to resist pressure, some less so.

What are the consequences of going through testing like amniocentesis—consequences for the woman, even when the results come back as desired? The pregnancy in its first half becomes overshadowed by the concern for what might happen during the second: If the possibility exists that her pregnancy may be leading not to a baby but to an abortion because of a "genetic defect," the woman's experience of the pregnancy, the fetus, and of her own motherhood is profoundly affected. For many of the women I interviewed, a new state of pregnancy had been constructed: a pregnancy without a baby. The effects were an awesome silence from a belly growing larger—a belly to be hidden in big sweaters, not flaunted in maternity clothes. The fear of having to become the executioner of one's hopes meant that any early movement of the fetus that was felt became denied, acknowledgment of the sensation of movement was delayed, the quickening slowed, awaiting a phone call.

What are the consequences of learning fetal sex, an often unasked question answered? Well, in many cases, perhaps not what one would expect. Certainly the sexual stereotyping that follows is of no surprise: boys kick, are strong and vigorous; girls squirm, are gentle, lively. But the effect on the mother is not what studies of son preference would lead one to expect: boys are conceptualized as other, different, separate—their mothers, to their own surprise, are disappointed. Girls, on the other hand, are considered part of a mother's self, are welcome. Mona Lisa, it would seem, had just learned it was a girl.

What are the consequences of learning bad news? (Indeed, what is the definition of bad news?) The news is overwhelming. Too many dimensions need to be considered all at once: length of life, quality of life, physical abilities, mental abilities. Factors one person may find as decisive, another finds as ambiguous. To decide what kind of life is worth bringing into the world is to decide the meaning of life—and by tomorrow. A decision has to be made; in some cases a moving fetus has to be stilled, and quickly. When news is bad, it is very, very bad—much worse than I ever expected. Women use the language of murder, of infanticide. The responsibility is awesome: sparing your child from its life. Here is a grief that should move the world; but the grief gets silenced, trivialized. The keening of mothers has never made much difference in our world.

That, in 1986, is about where matters stood in my study of the tentative pregnancy. But the book had a subtitle and a subtext: Prenatal Diagnosis and the Future of Motherhood. This technology has consequences, I was convinced, not just for the relatively small number of women who were at that moment being defined as "at high risk," nor even for the increasingly high percentage of women who will in the future be defined as at risk as the technology becomes more widespread and ripples out, but for all pregnancies and for all who will mother. Genetic technology changes the very way in which we think about pregnancy. And here I find the satisfaction of the "I told you so" at its grimmest. There is no pleasure to be had in having seen where all of this was heading.

The conventional wisdom—the male-dominated, patriarchally focused wisdom—worried about prenatal diagnosis and selective abortion as either a type of, or a forerunner to, an acceptable form of euthanasia. If we don't draw the line here at the fetus, people argued, where will we draw the line? Conversely, but from the same underlying perspective, some people argued that prenatal diagnosis was a valuable technology, sparing the fetus the anguish of potential existence under unbearable conditions. The argument then slowly shifted to a discussion of what conditions are unbearable, and just what makes them unbearable. To a large extent the discussion was, and is, a valuable and informative one. What makes that wisdom patriarchally focused, however (whether it comes out of the mouths and pens of men *or* women philosophers, activists, bioethicists, physicians, or genetic counselors), is that it puts the fetus at the center of all arguments. The only question addressed becomes: Are we behaving in the best interests of the fetus?

I spoke to women in my study. I looked at the costs to women. It has been very difficult for many people who have read my work to understand that focus. So what, they ask me, are the long-term consequences of the tentative pregnancy on "bonding" and infant development? The assumption, the bottom line of their argument, is that if something has no consequences for the child, no consequences exist. Genetic technology has consequences. It changes women's experience of pregnancy. The use of this technology—of all the varied technologies of prenatal diagnosis and selective abortion and now of selective implantation—reconstructs pregnancy in men's image.

What *is* pregnancy? This question lies at the heart of understanding the consequences of both prenatal diagnosis and the rapidly developing technologies of procreation. For women, pregnancy is a slow process of separation; part of us goes on to become someone else. The whole, the totality that is self—at first slowly, with a flutter, a rumble, a movement from within, and then suddenly and dramatically at the moment of birth as part of ourselves comes out through ourselves, as some*thing* held inside becomes some*one* held outside—that totality shatters into two parts.

What happens when we use the vantage point of men to describe this experience of women? Reality is turned on its head. Babies are "expected" and then "delivered," packages from outside. Babies "arrive," they "enter the world." And most insidiously of all, we "bond" with them—as if when the cord was cut, two became one, not one became two. Women do not feel babies arrive; we feel them *leave*. For us, birth is not a moment of attachment; it is a moment of separation.

Compounding the conflicting definitions of pregnancy and childbirth is a technology that further separates the baby from its mother—it separates the baby from the pregnancy. Conceptually, the fetus becomes a potential patient to be tested; visually, the free-floating fetus, made visible by its mother being rendered invisible, enters public awareness; and physically, a preimplantation diagnosis manipulates the material that will become the baby in a procedure conducted outside of the woman's body. The technology we have developed and continue to develop reifies a male notion of pregnancy, of the making of babies. It assumes, and thus demands of women, that our experience parallel men's, that we (like men) start from separation and come (and only with caution) to intimacy.

So what is pregnancy? For men, the focus is on the seed, the material that will become the baby. Even if we are belatedly recognized also as producers of seed, women still remain the place where men's seed grows. The seed is essential, considered determinative; the place it grows is considered a variable. Seeds are culled, sorted, graded, evaluated. The good ones are to be planted, to be given space to grow. Women are merely the space.

Pregnancy thus becomes, when constructed from a patriarchal focus, a production process, the transformation of seed to baby. The effects of that way of thinking are now coming to haunt us: as pregnant women are increasingly subjected to social control, we are seeing what looks very much like the regulation of untrusted, unskilled workers. And as a process of production, pregnancy becomes a service, the service ultimately becoming available for purchase. Surrogacy has become a thinkable thought; pregnant women are no longer necessarily the mothers of the children they carry within. Less a transformation of self, pregnancy has become a contractual agreement. It is to some extent, perhaps, an agreement between a woman and a man, but more fundamentally, it is an agreement between a woman and some genetic material. Thus, in effect it is an agreement between a woman and the controllers of that material— the father, the state, or the (purchasing) potential adopters.

The technology we develop grows out of this constructed contractual way of thinking, this perception of babies not as growing out of their mothers, flesh of their flesh, part of their lives, bodies, and communities, but as separate beings implanted within. The technology then reifies the ideology as we develop methods that allow us to create separate beings in test tubes, choosing which to implant. Preimplantation diagnosis is being offered as the coming alternative to prenatal diagnosis, and women may eventually come to be seen as just one possible site for implantation.

It is thus important to understand that this technology of prenatal diagnosis, and the specific technology of amniocentesis, does not come about in a vacuum. It develops in the context of all of the new reproductive technologies, including those that arrived with much fanfare such as in vitro fertilization and embryo transfer treatments for infertility. Amniocentesis has crept in more quietly, but it is part of the whole, occurring in a context in which women are more and more being seen as sites for fetal growth or, worse yet, barriers to fetal care.

An additional point of context is the fact that the technology is also developing in the midst of a major turn toward nature in the never-ending nature versus nurture debate. Articles about the genetic bases for the human condition appear weekly now. The search for "the gene for" anything and everything is on. In the past year there have been articles about the genetic bases for cancer, homosexuality, low birth weight, criminal behavior, altruism, and math scores. Recently a student of mine brought in a clipping: "Study suggests a genetic predisposition to divorce" read the headline, but the reassuring subhead countered: "The genetic effect would not doom people to divorce, researchers said." Here was the *New York Post*'s report of yet another twin study.

As any geneticist could explain, it is, of course, a far too simplistic vision of the way genes work. Genes don't "cause" divorce or cancer; genes interact with environments—the internal environment of the body, and the external social and political environments in which that body moves. But the image of a gene for particular characteristics, from alcoholism to sainthood, seems to persist. Some argue that it persists because it is actively constructed. Hubbard and Wald in *Exploding the Gene Myth* (1993) give an example of four newspaper articles in the *Boston Globe* on a single day: "Genetic link hinted in smoking cancers"; "Schizophrenia gene remains elusive"; "A gene that causes pure deafness"; and "Do the depressed bring on problems?" The article on "the depressed" relies on studies of twins the researchers believed to be "prone" to depression, finding that the more depressed twins had had more traumatic events, such as rape, assault, being fired from a job, and so forth. Because the depression was assumed to be genetic, the traumatic events were assumed to have been "brought on" by the depressed women themselves. Those of you who think that being raped or assaulted might cause the depression clearly are not thinking in genetically sophisticated terms.

The schizophrenia article isn't much better. Yet again, a gene for schizophrenia cannot be found, and yet again the article quotes a psychologist reassuring the public that the gene is there somewhere, just not yet found. The smoking article is perhaps the most interesting: it seems (it's *hinted*) that some people might carry a gene that makes them especially vulnerable to smoking-related cancers. If the gene exists, and the article says that there is only a "hint" of a "link" to such a gene, the researcher estimates that 52% of the population may have it: more than half of us are particularly vulnerable to cancer from smoking; the rest are just ordinarily vulnerable. Thus 48% of the population should not smoke and 52% of the population *really* shouldn't smoke.

The study cited about deafness is the only solid study of the four. A gene relating their deafness was indeed found among the members of one extended family in Costa Rica. Typically, this would not be a newsworthy story in Boston; but, as Hubbard and Wald point out, it gives substance to the other stories: See, there is a "gene for" things. We just have to keep looking for that gene for getting raped, or becoming schizophrenic, or getting cancer from smoking.

What has this to do with amniocentesis and prenatal diagnosis? As the hunt for the "gene for" goes on, the primary population having their genes tested often appears to be fetuses. Genetic testing in amniocentesis, and in the related test of chorionic villi sampling, is supposed to tell us if the fetus has the gene for various conditions. As the realm of problems that are believed to be genetically grounded expands, the problems for which fetuses can be tested also expands.

All of this speculation is gaining ground as the environmental causes of illness, disability, and death grow both larger and more clear. Our scientists and our newspapers focus not outside but inside, looking not at class, but at chromosomes; they look not at pollution indicators, but at genetic markers. New York City declares it has no money to provide antibiotics for homeless children with earaches, while in the same week the *New York Times* carries an article telling of the wonderful breakthroughs being made in diagnosing the genetic markers for deafness. The deaf community signs its anguish and goes unheard.

It is in the midst of all this that trumpets sound the great fanfare to welcome the newest and biggest and best scientific project yet: mapping the human genome. The earth mapped and conquered, space well charted, the scientists turn to internal frontiers. It is not just the major chromosomal disorders, not just a few dreadful diseases they seek to pinpoint; they want the whole story.

The little bits of information will be offered by clinicians, by genetic counselors, by geneticists, and physicians to pregnant women. Genetic information, like all fortune-telling, works in probabilities, possibilities, and potentials. I see a tall dark stranger in your future: make of it what you will. I see an increased probability, on the order of 12%, of cardiovascular disease in your child when he reaches middle age: make of it what you will. Women anguish over the decision to terminate a pregnancy after a diagnosis of Down syndrome; after all, who can tell what degree of retardation the baby might have? Who can tell what physical problems it might have? Women anguish over these questions and then virtually all decide they cannot knowingly go through with it—they cannot deliberately bring a child into the world knowing what they know, however limited, about what the child would face. Women now will be given the bits, dribs and drabs, of partial information genetic decoding will offer—an increased chance of this, risk of that, probability of the other. Based on this information they will be asked to decide whether to terminate a pregnancy.

Genetic and medical information is never enough. Just as women have had to look not only at Down syndrome itself, but at what our society offers in its institutions, services, and support for people with Down syndrome in order to make their decisions, so too will women now have to look not just at increased risks of, say, cancer, but at increased use of cancer-causing materials. These decisions of whether to continue or to terminate a pregnancy are never "medical" decisions. They are social decisions.

Increased knowledge, without increased responsibility on the part of the society, translates to increased knowledge with the inevitable burden of responsibility on mothers. We are asking mothers to become the gatekeepers of life. We are individualizing social problems of disease and disability, medicalizing life itself, and doing it through the bellies of pregnant women.

I find the language of individual choice untenable in this situation. Women are asked to "choose" whether to bring a child with certain genetic predispositions into the world, but they are not given choices about the environment in which that child would live. When a women "chooses" aborting rather than bringing to birth a child with a particular condition or predisposition, she is doing so in a world that sets the parameters of that child's life just as surely as genes do. Abortion can be the right choice, the moral choice, the only choice, but it, like birthing the child, is always a choice in a context.

When bioethicists debate reproductive choices and issues,

when Supreme Court justices think about them, they are understood to be the great moral issues of our time. When pregnant women face these choices they are defined in terms of
"anxiety." Virtually all of the medical research on the social and
psychological consequences of prenatal diagnosis continues to
be couched in the language of anxiety. It is as if what the woman
experiences awaiting the results of her amniocentesis is essentially the same emotion she experienced in seventh grade before
a math test. And when she chooses an abortion, her reaction is
most usually measured in terms of "depression."

I remember the first time I presented this research to a group
of physicians. It was at a continuing medical education seminar
held in Aspen. (They fit in some lectures early in the morning
and then late in the evening, après-ski.) At 10 PM I was telling a
group of doctors, legs stretched out, tanned faces gleaming
with the day's sun, about how the women suffered when they
aborted, following prenatal diagnosis. As I spoke, the legs
pulled in; the men sat up. They got angry and began to argue.
"My women," one said, "my women never felt anything like
that. They are *grateful*. They have their abortions and then they
have another baby." I thought of the women I had interviewed,
of some of the cruel things they told me doctors had thought-
lessly said or done, and of their silence with their doctors. I
thought, who would have the nerve to cry in front of this man,
open grief up to him? Later, one of the wives came up to me.
She had had a miscarriage a few years ago—just an ordinary
miscarriage—but it had all come back to her as I spoke. Of
course these poor women grieved and suffered, and, she continued, if her husband hadn't understood her grief, how could he
have understood that of his patients?

Later, as technology for earlier diagnosis became more
widely available, the climate began to shift. Now there was
some openness to hearing about how hard later diagnosis
was. Once chorionic villi sampling had become more widely
available, once early amniocentesis had made results possible
before the fourteenth week of pregnancy, the doctors suddenly changed their tune: late abortions are indeed traumatic;
the old amniocentesis was indeed a problem. As is so often
the case, having a solution enables people to recognize, or at

least to acknowledge, a problem. And early prenatal diagnosis does indeed help solve some of the problems of later prenatal diagnosis.

But I have to remember, too, a phone call I got one evening. A woman had tracked me down at home after having read my book. I got a fair number of such calls just after *The Tentative Pregnancy* was published. This woman told her tale—a tale I had grown to know quite well. She had had her abortion and gone right back to work. She was a physician, as a matter of fact. And then one afternoon a couple of weeks later, she couldn't take it anymore. She just started crying out of nowhere. Leaving the office and walking for hours, she found herself wandering in a bookstore at one point and, oddly enough, found my book. Standing in the store, she cried, recognizing herself and her grief in these women. She took a couple of months off, allowed herself time to recover from her loss, allowed herself to understand her loss as real, genuine, and worthy of grief rather than purely of gratitude. She thanked me, I thanked her, and just before she hung up, she said, "And think how much worse it would have been with an amniocentesis." "What?" "Oh," she said, "hadn't I mentioned? I had a chorionic villi sampling, and my abortion was at ten weeks."

Some say that doing testing earlier on will make the experience easier. It simply has to, doesn't it? And studies of women who have chosen earlier diagnostic techniques do indicate that the earlier techniques, even with higher risks of causing miscarriage, are chosen precisely because earlier abortions are supposed to be—are expected to be—less difficult (Kolker, 1990; Wertz, 1990; Zimmerman, 1989; Kolker, 1993). But just as a late abortion following amniocentesis might be easier and preferable to, say, euthanasia on an infant, and still be a tragedy in its own right, so too might an earlier abortion be easier than a later one, but still be experienced as tragic. We don't have to do a calculus of pain. This is, however, a technology founded on a calculus of pain, grief, and tragedy. It introduces that calculus into each woman's pregnancy. However one feels about abortion, whatever one sees as the consequence of all this testing for fetuses, the technology of prenatal diagnosis has changed and continues to change women's experience of pregnancy.

People will continue to be born with and to develop abilities and disabilities, strengths and weaknesses, resources and vulnerabilities. I do not really believe that those aspects of life will change, no matter how much mapping one does of chromosomal territory. But mothers will suffer and motherhood will have changed. That has consequences. That is of consequence.

ACKNOWLEDGMENTS

A version of this chapter appears as the introduction to the 1993 edition of *The Tentative Pregnancy* (W. W. Norton).

BIBLIOGRAPHY

HUBBARD, R., & Wald, E. (1993). *Exploding the gene myth.* Boston: Beacon.

KOLKER, A. (1993). Chorionic villus sampling. In B. K. Rothman (Ed.), *The encyclopedia of childbearing: Critical perspectives* (pp. 74–75). Phoenix: Oryx.

KOLKER, A., Burke, B. M., & Phillips, J. U. (1990). Attitudes about abortion of women who undergo prenatal diagnosis. In D. Wertz (Ed.), *Research in the sociology of health care* (pp. 49–73).

ROTHMAN, B. K. (1986). *The tentative pregnancy: Prenatal diagnosis and the future of motherhood.* New York: Viking. New edition: (1993). *The tentative pregnancy: How amniocentesis changes the experience of motherhood.* New York: Norton.

ZIMMERMAN, D. M. (1989). *Women's Experience with Chorionic Villus Sampling.* Unpublished master's thesis, Yale University School of Nursing, New Haven, CT.

14 Reproductive Genetic Testing and Pregnancy Loss:

The Experience of Women

RITA BECK BLACK

Introduction

A woman who undergoes prenatal genetic testing—whether it be chorionic villi sampling, amniocentesis, ultrasound, maternal serum alpha-fetoprotein testing, or whatever the current technology serves up—experiences many physical and psychological changes during her pregnancy. Chances are high that this is a "wanted pregnancy," but the meaning of that phrase may be clouded by issues of genetic risk or by any prior reproductive difficulties she may have had. We do not know very much about the potential or developing relationship between mother and fetus when it occurs against the backdrop of genetic risk. We as yet, for example, know little about how the experience of pregnancy is altered when the woman sees the baby on ultrasound or sees the baby's chromosomes and learns its sex (Black, 1992; Blumberg, 1984; Fletcher, 1972).

When pregnancy loss follows genetic testing, a woman faces in rapid succession two major and contrasting life crises: pregnancy and death. The following discussion of the psychological experiences of women undergoing prenatal genetic testing thus begins with a review of the common human experiences of loss and pregnancy loss before moving on to consider the more particularized experience of pregnancy loss following prenatal genetic testing. Results from a study of pregnancy loss among women who had undergone amniocentesis or chorionic villi sampling (CVS) will be presented to provide a detailed illustration of women's experiences and to highlight needed directions for future research inquiries.

Loss and Bereavement

The wide variations in people's individual responses to bereavement (Osterweis, Solomon, & Green, 1984; Wortman & Silver, 1989) suggest the need for considerable caution in developing any assessments about what are normal or usual behaviors or feelings of a person who loses a loved one. Certainly such cautions must be applied in any research efforts to assess women's experiences after pregnancy loss. Most descriptions of the bereavement process (Osterweis et al., 1984) outline a series of general phases through which many people pass, with recognition that some people will experience relatively mild distress while others will show persistent difficulties for a prolonged period of time (Wortman & Silver, 1989). However, the lack of consensus about criteria for distinguishing normal from abnormal grief suggests that concepts about the phases of the bereavement process should be used only as a loose framework for predicting or assessing any bereaved individual's experiences.

For the same reasons, it is difficult to define when recovery should occur or even whether the concept of recovery has meaning in this context. The quality and quantity of reactions over time seem more important than a precise endpoint in time in assessing the normality of a grief process (Osterweis et al., 1984). Concern seems appropriate when the bereaved person continues, even some months after the loss has occurred, to lack any hope for the future, or shows a worrisome intensity of anger, self-blame, or depression. Chronic grief should be suspected when there is not only sadness but also "active resistance to changing that feeling. Not only is there no movement [in that person's life], but there also is a sense that the person will not permit any movement" (Osterweis et al., 1984, p. 54).

This is not to say that favorable resolutions of the grief process mean a return to life just as it was before the loss. "People do adapt and stabilize, . . . [but] some of the pain of loss may remain for a lifetime" (Osterweis et al., 1984, p. 53). Certain events such as birthdays, anniversaries, or missed developmental milestones may be particularly powerful triggers of strong and painful emotions. However, the process of recovery would appear to be on the right course when the bereaved person seems able, despite occasional setbacks, to invest in current life, feel hopeful about the future, and experience some gratification from present activities.

Parental Bereavement

Although not all women who lose pregnancies, whether through elective termination or miscarriage, think of themselves as bereaved parents, clinical experience suggests that many women who undergo prenatal genetic testing do speak of the fetus as their baby and say they mourn the loss of that child if the pregnancy is lost. The literature on grief suggests that parents who lose a child face a particularly long and complicated bereavement course (Osterweis et al., 1984). Although they have much in common with other bereaved adults, bereaved parents also face several unique aspects in their grief (Rando, 1985). Perhaps foremost, the death of a child is "out of turn." Deaths of infants and children are no longer common events in families and thus our life-cycle expectations suggest that parents will die before their children. Social reactions to the death of a child are also often problematic. Other parents, in particular, may attach a certain social stigma to such losses because they become anxious about their own vulnerability to a similar loss.

Parents' potentially strongest sources of support, their spouses, are less available because each is deeply involved in his or her own grief. In reaction, feelings of anger and blame may be displaced onto the spouses because they are closest at hand. One spouse may negatively misinterpret the behavior of the other when the pace and style of their grieving differs. Sexual problems, too, may arise when one partner's grief blocks sexual feelings, while for the other partner sexual contact is seen as healing (Osterweis et al., 1984).

Other problems common to many forms of bereavement may become particularly hard to resolve when it is a child who has died. For example, the often-found anger toward the deceased may be especially hard to acknowledge and deal with when directed at a child. Parents must also "grow up with the loss" (Rando, 1985) as they note missed birthdays and major developmental milestones, while if there are other siblings, the parents must continue to function as parents, in the very role that they are trying to grieve for and relinquish.

Perhaps not surprising in view of these stresses are findings on the critical importance of the marital relationship in recovery after a child's death. The frequently different coping styles of mothers and fathers can become an increasing source of stress, although couples also may be drawn together as they share their common loss and develop understanding and respect for the differences in their coping styles (Glicken, Harmon, Siegel, & Rudd, 1986; Helmrath & Steinitz, 1978; Jones et al., 1984; LaRoche et al., 1984; Osterweis et al., 1984; Peppers & Knapp, 1980; Rosenblatt & Burns, 1986; Videka-Sherman, 1987; Videka-Sherman & Lieberman, 1985).

Family and friends are often important sources of initial support and frequently are the only people, apart from spouses, from whom help is sought. However, even close relatives can become less available and sympathetic over time. Parents often report that others expect them to "snap out of it" or "get back to normal" when the parents still feel a need to mourn and talk about their loss (Glicken et al., 1986; Helmrath & Steinitz, 1978; Videka-Sherman, 1987).

Pregnancy Loss

The woman who begins a pregnancy only to lose it, whatever the reason, finds herself aboard a rollercoaster of changing emotions and coping tasks. Pregnancy itself has been described as a "critical phase" in a woman's life (Blum, 1980), precipitating one of life's normal, developmental crises (Erikson, 1950). It often is a time when a woman reconsiders her previous roles, coping strategies, and self-image (Bibring, 1959; Bibring, Dwyer, Huntington, & Valenstein, 1961; Deutsch, 1945).

Physical and emotional change occur over the course of gestation, with the conclusion of pregnancy, regardless of timing or outcome, requiring additional psychological and physiological adjustments (Blumberg, 1984).

Miscarriage

Unfortunately, the same tradition that viewed the mother's bonding with the baby as developing only gradually, accelerating at the time of quickening (Bibring et al., 1961; Blumberg, 1984), influenced thinking about early miscarriage as a "nonevent" (Osterweis et al., 1984) and minimized the personal anguish generated by early pregnancy losses. In contrast, a "woman-centered view of pregnancy" (Rothman, 1989), suggests that the woman's construction of the meaning of her pregnancy will influence profoundly her experience of its loss.

The woman who finds herself unexpectedly pregnant and does not want to be pregnant, in effect may choose not to enter into a relationship with that fetus (and, in fact, may prefer to use the term fetus rather than baby). The fact of its loss may not evoke psychological feelings of grief in that woman for that particular pregnancy. In contrast, a woman may embrace her relationship with the baby (and prefer to say baby rather than fetus) from the earliest moment she is aware of her pregnancy. Its loss, regardless of gestation, will evoke grief, the nature of which will be colored by the motivations for the pregnancy (Kessler, 1979) and the nature of the relationship that had been formed.

Miscarriage thus may call an abrupt halt to the woman's thinking about herself as a mother and to fantasizing about her future life with a child. If siblings have been told about the new brother or sister, parents face the task of finding words to explain miscarriage, genetic defects, or pregnancy termination. Additional hardships include having to inform friends, family, and perhaps employers about the loss. Or alternatively, if the loss occurred very early in gestation, the woman and her partner may have told almost no one else about the pregnancy. In such cases, they face either a very lonely struggle with their grief or the difficult role of informing significant others about the pregnancy at the same time they tell them of its loss. The privacy of an early pregnancy loss thus makes it more difficult for them to receive the social support that may prove helpful in facilitating their bereavement process (Vachon et al., 1982).

Research findings have begun to confirm women's statements about the anguish of miscarriage. At least some women and their partners experience the volatile emotions and feelings of shock, disorganization, guilt, and loss similar to the bereavement reactions seen after other significant losses. One study (Neugebauer et al., 1992), for example, reports a three-fold increase in depressive symptoms in the six months following miscarriage. These findings are particularly powerful because the study was unique in drawing from a large sample of 382 miscarrying women who were interviewed at two weeks, six weeks, or six months after loss.

Factors thought to affect the heightened distress felt after pregnancy or perinatal loss include the following: loss of a wanted pregnancy; loss at a later stage of gestation; poorer overall physical health; poorer quality of marital relationship; and higher level of mental health difficulties before the loss occurred (Toedter, Lasker, & Alhadeff, 1988). Incongruent grieving among couples and stress on the marital relationship may be negative consequences of a pregnancy loss when the man's process of attachment to the child is not as developed as that of the mother's at the time of the loss (Peppers & Knapp, 1980).

Elective Termination of Pregnancy

At first glance, the decision to electively terminate a pregnancy might appear to have little in common with the spontaneous, uncontrollable end of a pregnancy through miscarriage. Indeed, the research literature on general, elective abortion consistently finds few significant emotional problems as a result of that procedure (Figa-Talamanca, 1981; Nadelson, 1978; Smith, 1973). However, a small percentage of women do suffer worrisome psychological reactions after elective terminations. Among those at increased risk are women with abnormal obstetrical histories, medical indications for the abortion, or negative or ambivalent attitudes toward abortion (Ashton, 1980; Figa-Talamanca, 1981). Viewed another way, the literature suggests that women who want to develop a relationship with the baby, or whose ambivalence prevents them from blocking the development of that relationship, are vulnerable to strong reactions after a termination.

Prenatal Genetic Testing and Pregnancy Loss

Research on the experience of prenatal testing (most research on experience concerns amniocentesis) suggests that women feel heightened anxiety before the testing, worry as they await test results, and experience a decline in anxiety if they receive word that no abnormality has been detected (Adler, Keyes, & Robertson, 1991). The majority of those who already have children will tell at least one child in the family about the testing (Black & Furlong, 1984a, 1984b) and provide at least a partial explanation of pregnancy loss if the pregnancy is terminated after detection of a defect (Furlong & Black, 1984). Even very young children and those unaware of all the facts show reactions to their parents' distress and maternal absence when a pregnancy termination occurs after genetic testing (Furlong & Black, 1984). Younger children may have an especially hard time coping with complete information about the termination (Furlong & Black, 1984).

Some limited inquiry has also been made into the developing relationship between the mother and baby prior to amniocentesis. At least some women attempt to withhold investment in the pregnancy until test results are available (Beeson & Golbus, 1979). These are the "tentative" pregnancies (Rothman, 1986) in which women try to delay use of maternity clothing and to deny awareness of the baby's movement until testing has been completed.

However, CVS and early ultrasonography create a psychological milestone of quickening in the first trimester. Rather than feeling the baby kick, the woman (and perhaps the father) sees its heart beat and its limbs move. For the woman at risk for a serious defect in the baby, the technology itself works against any efforts she may have made to maintain an emotional distance until results are confirmed (Black, 1992; Blumberg, 1984; Milne & Rich, 1981). She remains physiologically in the more unsettling period of first trimester symptoms and changes, while psychologically being propelled rapidly forward. Thus,

from the outset, we can predict that women undergoing terminations of wanted pregnancies after CVS or amniocentesis will
be more likely to face a more difficult emotional course.

Decision-making after a defect is detected can itself be a major source of stress and anguish for women and their partners
(Blumberg, 1984; Rothman, 1986). Although on one level
women choose the testing with full knowledge that they might
face the need to decide about continuing the pregnancy, on another level they often remain optimistic about beating the odds,
however high they may be, and coming out on the winning side
of the technology.

The prognostic implications of the specific defect that is
found can also have a significant impact on decision-making
(Blumberg, 1984). For example, although the woman may have
come for testing because of concern about higher risks for
Down syndrome, the test might reveal a clinically ambiguous
abnormality. Chromosomal mosaicisms (where only a portion
of cells show chromosome abnormalities), new (de novo) chromosome rearrangements, or unclear details on the ultrasound
picture are some of the findings with uncertain clinical significance. Other specific disorders, such as those involving the
sex chromosomes, may be identified. Such disorders may carry
some, but by no means certain, risks for lowered intelligence,
learning problems, or behavioral difficulties.

A number of authors have described the anguish of terminating a pregnancy in the second trimester, after amniocentesis
(Ashery, 1977; Blumberg, Golbus, & Hanson, 1975; Donnai,
Charles, & Harris, 1981; Fletcher, 1972; Furlong & Black, 1984;
Jones et al., 1984). Parents often report mild to moderate depression for at least the first few months after the losses, with
mothers, more often than fathers, reporting that they find it
difficult to feel that the incident is behind them (Jones et al.,
1984). Since, in previous years, these later terminations involved a procedure all too similar to labor and delivery, the particular stresses surrounding these termination procedures has
been a major focus of concern and some medical centers have
made efforts to develop protocols for the sensitive handling of
such terminations (Magyari, Wedehase, Ifft, & Callahan, 1987).

The increased use of dilation and evacuation techniques

(D&E) for later terminations avoids such concerns because the termination is done under general anesthesia. However, some professionals have pointed out that the process of delivering the baby and the option to see and perhaps hold it carry the psychological value of confirming the loss and thereby facilitating grieving (Magyari et al., 1987).

Pregnancy Loss after CVS or Amniocentesis: A Closer Look

The literature discussed above provides a framework for considering a research project conducted by the author on pregnancy loss among women who had undergone CVS or amniocentesis. Findings from prior research on pregnancy loss and prenatal testing has been limited by very small sample sizes and retrospective reporting. The project presented here is unique in its access to a large, national sample and in its access to women in the months immediately following their pregnancy losses. Review of the findings presented herein also highlights both the value and the limitations of using structured, quantitative research methodologies of large samples to learn about women's experiences.

Subjects were obtained from the women enrolled in the National Institute of Child Health and Human Development's collaborative chorionic villus sampling and amniocentesis study (Rhoads et al., 1989), and were those who experienced pregnancy losses as a result of either elective terminations after abnormal test results or spontaneous abortions. The overall participation rate was 60.5%. The 121 women in the pregnancy loss study were mainly white (94%), married (91%), well educated (63% had completed college or a more advanced level of education), and affluent (74% had family incomes of $40,000 or more). (Additional details about recruitment procedures and demographic characteristics of the sample are provided in Black [1989].) It is important to note that the lack of diversity in the sample mirrored a similar deficiency in the larger collaborative study and many previous research projects. Women of color and from lower socioeconomic groups generally did not have equal access to CVS at the time of the project (the mid-1980s), and the general lack of equal access to genetic services continues to be a significant problem (Paul & Kavanaugh, 1990). The importance of future research studies involving diverse populations is discussed later in this chapter.

Subjects participated in semi-structured telephone interviews and completed mailed questionnaires at approximately one to two months after the pregnancy loss and then again at approximately six months after the loss. Each participant completed by mail the Profile of Mood States (POMS) (McNair, Lorr, & Droppelman, 1971), which provided an assessment of their general level of mood disturbance after the losses. They also completed by mail the Dyadic Adjustment Scale (DAS) (Spanier, 1976), which asks questions about the general functioning of their major relationship (usually marriage for the women in this study). Interviews were tape recorded with the consent of the participant. (More complete details about instrumentation and findings are available in Black [1989, 1991, 1992].)

On one level, this project sought to confirm the already available evidence that pregnancy losses of prenatal diagnosis patients often precipitate a grief process. The literature on parental and other forms of bereavement suggested there would be considerable variation in the women's grief levels, although generally a greater degree of distress at the first interview, with perhaps some easing by the six month contact. It also was hypothesized that more difficult grief reactions would be found among the women who had losses later in their pregnancies; had a greater number of prior miscarriages; had previously had a pregnancy in which the baby carried a serious defect; had some known genetic risks; were older; had used professional mental health services before the loss; and who perceived less emotional support from their partner, family, friends, and significant others.

Confirmation of these hypotheses would indicate that prenatal diagnosis patients who lose their pregnancies have much in common with others who lose children or loved ones. However, perhaps more important than confirming such likely similarities was learning more about what is unique in the bereavement experiences of women undergoing new forms of prenatal diagnostic technologies. Since an explicit aim of the project was to provide information to guide the development of services for this population, the study sought to determine both the minimum level of supportive follow-up indicated for all prenatal diagnosis patients who lose pregnancies as well as variables for assessment to guide identification and treatment of women who could profit from more specialized assistance.

The pregnancy loss group's average mood level (POMS) at the first interview was poorer than that of the control group of pregnant prenatal diagnosis patients but showed significant improvement at the second interview (Black, 1989). Sixty-eight percent of the women said they were able to resume normal work and social activities by the end of the first month after the loss, with 80% reporting normal levels of activities at six months (Black, 1989). The majority said they received understanding and positive support from husbands, partners, and significant others, and average scores on the Dyadic Adjustment Scale were well within range reported by the scale's author for married couples (Black, 1989; Spanier, 1976).

These positive general findings for the majority, while encouraging, nonetheless should not divert attention from the greater difficulties experienced by minorities of the women or from the internal anguish some felt even as they functioned quite well in their daily lives. Indeed, the mood scores on the POMS showed very large standard deviations (Black, 1989), thus showing much more severe distress among some of the women. Similarly, in the ratings of social and work functioning, close to one-third of the women reported reduced functioning at the one month assessment and 21% still noted some decrement at six months (Black, 1989). Comparisons of the women's reports of support from partners and significant others revealed small, yet statistically significant declines in perceived support (Black, 1989, 1991).

A few key factors were found to be associated with the women's reported mood levels at the second interview (Black, 1989). Total POMS scores at one to two months after the loss (Time #1) and six months after the loss (Time #2) were strongly correlated ($r = 0.59$). Measures of post-loss social support most consistently showed associations with mood. Women who reported greater mood disturbance at Time #2 more often had sought some type of mental health services after the loss, described less support from and congruence with their partners at either Time #1 or #2 and reported less support from family and friends at either Time #1 or #2. The only pregnancy-related variable that emerged with a significant correlation was length of gestation, with women who had later losses reporting poorer mood at both Time #1 ($r = 0.20$) and #2 ($r = 0.17$).

Examination of the women's responses to two specific sections of the interview provides additional information on their experiences. First, a series of questions asked about the understanding and support the woman felt she was getting from her male partner (usually husband). (See Black [1991] for detailed discussion of the couples material.) As noted earlier, women did perceive a small, but statistically significant decline in partner support between the first and second interviews. Ratings of the overall impact of the loss on their relationships showed considerable variation at both interviews, with increased negativity at the second interview. Women reporting that they felt closer to their partner after the loss declined from 62% to 51%. Those reporting that they felt pulled more apart from their partner increased from 7% to 14%.

Later in this chapter I will consider the implications of those findings for development of minimum standards for psychosocial services for prenatal diagnosis patients who lose pregnancies. However, these general recommendations must be developed in the context of a more detailed look at the experiences behind the numbers. Themes identified in the women's open-ended comments about two aspects of their experiences will be presented: 1) the experience of pregnancy loss in the context of their relationships with husbands or male partners (Black, 1991); and 2) the experiences they described when asked how it had been to see the fetus on ultrasound (Black, 1992).

Physical Experience

The physical experience of the pregnancy and loss marked a central difference between the men and women. All the women, regardless of type of loss, experienced at least some pain, encounters with medical personnel, and a period of physical recovery. The men, even if very involved, were described as bystanders.

Degree and Duration of Distress

Many of the women felt they experienced greater distress after the loss than did the men. Particularly striking were reports of divergence in partners' feelings over time, as the men seemed more quickly to put the loss behind them. All too often the women also felt their partners did not share their resurgence of painful feelings at the due date, when the baby would have been born.

Expression of Feelings

The women often said their partners did not discuss their reactions to the loss. Even, in some instances, when the man seemed to be grieving intensely, the women seemed to prefer a verbally or physically more expressive coping style than did their male partners. However, women often noted that they limited their own expression of grief to private times. An apparently normal round of work and social activities might exist alongside long and tearful evenings.

Sexuality

The majority said they experienced no change or perhaps enhancement of their sexual relationships. However, sex for some became associated with pain and loss, making it hard to feel sexual. Sexual strains also arose over conflicting priorities about whether to try to have another baby as well as different views about their likelihood of success. Some women who were trying to achieve another pregnancy also reported that they lost the pleasure of having spontaneous sexual encounters motivated solely for pleasure.

Couples' Coping Patterns

The interaction of each woman's personal experience of the loss interacted with her partner's experience to yield what I have called a conjoint coping pattern. Any evaluation of these coping patterns of course must be made very tentatively, but for the sake of discussion, I have characterized them as "satisfactory" or "problematic."

Satisfactory patterns included:

1. mutual agreement to limit discussion of feelings

2. mutual acceptance of differences in coping styles

3. mutual sharing of feelings about the loss, sometimes leading to a general increase in communication about a range of feelings and concerns

Problematic patterns included:

1. woman perceives that the burden is on her to initiate any discussion of the loss

2. woman does not act on her desire to express feelings, citing need to protect partner from painful feelings

3. woman does not act on her desire to express feelings, citing potential or actual lack of responsiveness from partner

4. woman precipitates a "fight" in order to evoke response from partner

A second section of the interview concerned the experience of undergoing ultrasound. Although there was no significant statistical association between frequency of ultrasound and mood scores, 60% said that seeing the ultrasound image had made them feel closer to the fetus. Forty-four percent responded affirmatively when asked if seeing the fetus had made coping with the loss more difficult. Only 9% felt it had made coping any easier.

Again, qualitative analyses provide a look at the experiences behind the numbers. A number of major themes were identified.

The Reality of Seeing

For many, seeing the fetus on the ultrasound screen marked a "moment of acceptance that you were indeed pregnant." Intellectualization gave way at that moment of recognition. "It made it more than a concept; it made it what appeared to be a living thing." For some who had tried to distance themselves from the pregnancy because of the genetic risk, the ultrasound tended to reduce that distance: "all the precautions my husband and I had taken to protect our feelings just went right out the window."

Additional Anguish

One woman said the ultrasound was the worst part of the testing. Another vividly described "flashing" on the ultrasound image as she thought through her plans to terminate the pregnancy. Others said it had heightened their general grief over the loss. Some wished they had not seen the fetus and suggested women be given the option not to see the ultrasound. Another spoke of not seeing the image as inconceivable, despite the distress it caused her. She could not imagine not watching along with the professionals who were seeing her "child."

Benefits of Confronting Reality

How could something be so emotionally painful and yet carry some benefits? The women's responses suggested that they were struggling with this paradox. For some, the benefit seemed to derive from the pregnancy having been made more real. For example, one woman who miscarried saw the fetal heartbeat at an initial ultrasound (when CVS was postponed) and then no heartbeat two weeks later. She compared her experience to a previous miscarriage when she had had so many doubts about what had happened. Here the "concrete" evidence made it easier to cope with the loss. Some women seemed almost grateful that they had been forced to confront the realities of their pregnancies:

> I think it's important to see it . . . to confront it. . . . I would have been better off if I had really let myself think about it more. . . . I was trying to sort of come in through the back door, saying if I didn't think about it then the loss wouldn't be as bad as if I had thought about [it]. . . . I'm glad I saw it and I think women should see it so they know that there was a reason for all the things they were going through.

Discussion

Interpreting the findings of my own research and that of others sometimes yields one of those situations where people differ on whether the glass is half full or half empty. A positive reading is that most women who undergo prenatal genetic testing, even those who terminate their pregnancies after a fetal defect is found, cope well with the experience. Grief reactions after pregnancy losses, while painful, usually seem to follow an expected course of gradual improvement without professional intervention. Extensive counseling or therapy does not seem to be needed or wanted by most women (Black, 1989).

On the other hand, a second look at the data brings into view not only that minority who experience greater coping difficulties but also the difficult decisions and painful feelings faced by those who carry on with their usual, everyday routines. Prenatal genetic testing is a major psychological and social event for women—even more so if the testing reveals a serious defect in the baby. The accumulated evidence confirms that these new technologies have changed the experience of pregnancy as well as the experience of pregnancy loss. As the women attest, major changes and even painful experiences are not necessarily evaluated negatively. For example, some women I spoke with said that seeing the ultrasound image intensified their grief, but they recognized the healing power of confronting their loss without avoidance. Unfortunately, others seemed more shaken by their experiences and less able to see positive aspects of their encounters with genetic testing.

There is enough information on women's experiences to support development of minimum service standards for women who lose pregnancies after prenatal genetic testing. The overwhelming majority of women interviewed for my study wanted at least some follow-up. For most, this meant a follow-up telephone call and referral, as needed, to appropriate support groups and mental health professionals knowledgeable about pregnancy loss, genetic disorders, and prenatal technologies. A minimum service standard for prenatal genetic testing programs (Black, 1989) should include: 1) at least one follow-up telephone call to all prenatal diagnosis patients who lose pregnancies; 2) assessment of psychosocial distress and need for additional services by inquiry about the woman's mood, recent use of mental health services, satisfaction with emotional support she is receiving from her partner and significant others, and interest in referrals to support groups or professional counselors; and 3) preventive intervention by providing information about the considerable variation and sometimes persistence of grief reactions, possible differences between partners in reactions to the loss, and likelihood of decline in support from others that will feel premature to the woman.

Clinical priorities for mental health professionals who provide therapeutic services to couples should include helping them: 1) to identify the unique personal meanings of the loss for each of them, their perceptions of its reproductive implications, and their preferred coping styles; 2) to openly discuss any differences that may emerge; 3) to negotiate a mutually acceptable balance between expression and containment of feelings; and 4) to negotiate a mutually acceptable decision about whether to attempt a future pregnancy.

Future research on the psychosocial experience of reproductive genetic testing and pregnancy loss has many exciting directions to pursue. Some research questions follow directly from my own and other previous studies. For example, fathers' reactions throughout testing and after pregnancy loss need to be studied carefully, not only for the men's own sake but also because of their interactive impact on the women. Similarly, a family-focused research agenda should investigate the impact of prenatal genetic testing on the parents' other children and on communication between family members. Service research also is needed that examines the impact of various models of supportive contact for prenatal diagnosis patients before and after detection of a serious defect in the fetus (Elder & Laurence, 1991). If there is increased access to reproductive genetic technology for women of color and economic disadvantage, certainly we must ask again many of the questions addressed in previous studies that have been done largely with white, highly educated, and relatively affluent women.

It also is important to recognize that there is a limit to what we can learn from giving large numbers of patients standardized instruments and structured questionnaires. Nomothetic, quantitative research provides information that is very helpful in setting service priorities and identifying at-risk populations (for example, knowing that the majority of prenatal diagnosis patients who lose pregnancies do not need extensive counseling, but that services should be organized to make more intensive services available for the minority who need it). The clinician, however, seeks information to guide interventions with individuals. Having used nomothetic data to identify that a patient is at increased risk for coping difficulties, the clinician seeks to " 'beat the odds' by way of skillful intervention" (Roberts, 1989, p. 67). Idiographic, qualitative techniques are more likely to prove helpful in guiding clinical practice.

In the study of women encountering the new genetic reproductive technologies, this translates into intensive qualitative studies that ask epistemological questions about the meaning of those experiences for women. For example, in my research I found no statistical difference in mood levels between women who miscarried rather than terminated their pregnancies. Future research with larger samples might or might not confirm this finding. However, a general mood score will never tell us anything about the different meanings these two experiences carry for women or their male partners. It is not enough just to ask whether one type of loss evokes more or less distress than another.

Recent work by a number of feminist scholars may prove useful in providing frameworks for looking at prenatal diagnosis patients in new ways. While a comprehensive review of feminist writing on women and reproductive issues is beyond the scope of this paper, three examples should suffice to illustrate the potential contributions of this literature.

Rothman (1989), in her discussion of pregnancy as a physical and social relationship, suggests that a women may choose not to enter into the social part of the relationship. Because of this element of choice, "some abortions are easy, avoiding motherhood, while some are hard, ending motherhood" (p. 107). How does this concept of choosing to enter into a maternal relationship apply to women undergoing prenatal testing? We know these are mostly wanted pregnancies and that ultrasound may have heightened the reality of the fetus as baby. Yet many women choose to end the relationship through abortion when a serious defect is found. Is this avoiding or ending motherhood? What factors enter into the woman's choice to enter that relationship? For example, what are the woman's experiences and knowledge about physical and mental disabilities and available services (Ashe, 1989)?

Philosopher Sara Ruddick (1989) has observed that three demands constitute maternal work and shape what she calls "maternal thinking." They are the demands for preservation, growth, and social acceptability; "to be a mother is to be committed to meeting these demands by works of preservative love, nurturance, and training" (p. 17). Ruddick talks of woman's labor to protect and sustain her baby, and later, her child. Yet Ruddick introduces a perplexing notion for those involved with reproductive genetic technologies when she asserts that a "mother takes care of her *fetus* by taking care of herself" (p. 50, Ruddick's italics). We need to know about women's thinking as they contemplate prenatal genetic testing and ending a pregnancy when a serious defect is identified. Who are they protecting? Can Ruddick's ideas about maternal demands and thinking help us formulate new ways to learn from the women undergoing prenatal testing? Can the woman, early into her first pregnancy, be thought of as a mother? How is prenatal testing different when the woman is already a mother to children?

A third example of how feminist scholarship can contribute new research perspectives comes from the work of scholars such as Gilligan (1982) and Belenky, Clinchy, Goldberger, and Tarule (1986). They ask questions about how women develop ways of knowing and about the perspectives from which women draw conclusions about morality, truth, knowledge, and authority. Researchers in reproductive genetics might ask: How does the woman undergoing CVS evaluate whether she is doing the right or the wrong thing? How does the woman's resolution of this question influence her psychosocial reaction to genetic testing or pregnancy termination? The learning styles of some women may emphasize the place of "received knowledge," that is, listening to the voices of others while placing little value on their own voices. In contrast, other women grow into an awareness of the constructed nature of knowledge and of their central role in interpreting and evaluating all evidence (Belenky et al., 1986). How do these different ways of knowing shape women's responses to genetic reproductive technology? For example, consider the woman who is accustomed to following the advice of experts and lacks confidence in her ability to make her own decisions. How does she feel as she confronts the option of terminating her pregnancy when professionals and perhaps also husband and friends say they cannot tell her what she should do.

Additional work is needed to determine which, if any, of these possible lines of inquiry will bear fruit. However, more important than any specific research question is the importance of ongoing inquiry into the meanings of genetic reproductive technologies for women. Psychosocial responses occur in context, and the context of genetic technologies is changing constantly as new technical options appear and as the very idea of genetic testing becomes woven into our social thread.

ACKNOWLEDGMENTS

The main study reported on in this paper was aided by a subcontract to Yale University Grant #HD19872, National Institute of Child Health and Human Development.

BIBLIOGRAPHY

ADLER, N. E., Keyes, S., & Robertson, P. (1991). Psychological issues in new reproductive technologies: Pregnancy-inducing technology and diagnostic screening. In J. Rodin & A. Collins (Eds.), *Women and new reproductive technologies: Medical, psychosocial, legal, and ethical dilemmas* (pp. 111–133). Hillsdale, NJ: Lawrence Erlbaum.

ASHE, A. (1989). Reproductive technology and disability. In S. Cohen & N. Taub (Eds.), *Reproductive laws for the 1990s* (pp. 69–124). Clifton, NJ: Humana Press.

ASHERY, R. S. (1977). Prenatal diagnosis: Is amniocentesis a crisis situation? In W. T. Hall & C. L. Young (Eds.), *Genetic disorders and social service interventions*. Pittsburgh: University of Pittsburgh Graduate School of Public Health.

ASHTON, J. R. (1980). The psychosocial outcomes of induced abortion. *British Journal of Obstetrics and Gynecology, 87,* 1115–1122.

BEESON, D., & Golbus, M. (1979). Anxiety engendered by amniocentesis. *Birth Defects: Original Article Series, XV*(5C), 191–197.

BELENKY, M. F., Clinchy, B. M., Goldberger, N. R., & Tarule, J. M. (1986). *Women's ways of knowing.* New York: Basic Books.

BIBRING, G. L. (1959). Some considerations of the psychological processes in pregnancy. *Psychoanalytic Study of the Child, 14,* 113–121.

BIBRING, G. L., Dwyer, T. F., Huntington, D. S., & Valenstein, A. F. (1961). A study of the psychological processes in pregnancy and of the earliest mother-child relationship. *Psychoanalytic Study of the Child, 16,* 9–27.

BLACK, R. B. (1989). A one and six month follow-up of prenatal diagnosis patients who lost pregnancies. *Prenatal Diagnosis, 9,* 795–804.

BLACK, R. B. (1991). Women's voices after pregnancy loss: Couples' patterns of communication and support. *Social Work in Health Care, 16,* 19–36.

BLACK, R. B. (1992). Seeing the baby: The impact of ultrasound technology. *Journal of Genetic Counseling, 1,* 45–54.

BLACK, R. B., & Furlong, R.M. (1984a). Impact of prenatal diagnosis in families. *Social Work in Health Care, 9,* 37–50.

BLACK, R. B., & Furlong, R. M. (1984b). Prenatal diagnosis: The experience in families who have children. *American Journal of Medical Genetics, 19,* 729–739.

BLUM, B. L. (1980). *Psychological aspects of pregnancy, birthing, and bonding.* New York: Human Sciences Press.

BLUMBERG, B. D. (1984). The emotional implications of prenatal diagnosis. In A. E. H. Emery & I. Pullen (Eds.), *Psychological aspects of genetic counseling* (pp. 201–217). New York: Academic Press.

BLUMBERG, B. D., Golbus, M. S., & Hanson, K. H. (1975). The psychological sequelae of abortion for a genetic indication. *American Journal of Obstetrics and Gynecology, 122,* 799–808.

DEUTSCH, H. (1945). *The psychology of women. Vol II.* New York: Grune & Stratton.

DONNAI, P., Charles, N., & Harris, R. (1981). Attitudes of patients after "genetic" termination of pregnancy. *British Medical Journal, 282,* 621–622.

ELDER, S. H., & Laurence, K. M. (1991). The impact of supportive intervention after second trimester termination of pregnancy for fetal abnormality. *Prenatal Diagnosis, 11,* 47–54.

ERIKSON, E. H. (1950). *Childhood and Society.* New York: Norton.

FIGA-TALAMANCA, I. (1981). Abortion and mental health. In J. E. Hodgson (Ed.), *Abortion and sterilization: Medical and social aspects* (pp. 181–208). New York: Academic Press.

FLETCHER, J. (1972). The brink: The parent-child bond in the genetic revolution. *Theological Studies, 33,* 457–485.

FURLONG, R. M., & Black, R. B. (1984). Pregnancy termination for genetic indications: The impact on families. *Social Work in Health Care, 10*, 17–34.

GILLIGAN, C. (1982). *In a different voice: Psychological theory and women's development.* Cambridge, MA: Harvard University Press.

GLICKEN, A. D., Harmon, R. J., Siegel, R. E., & Rudd, S. H. (1986). Maternal grieving following neonatal loss: A research study to guide clinical practice. In R. S. Pacholski (Ed.), *Researching death: Selected essays in death education and counseling* (pp. 103–114). Lakewood, OH: Forum for Death Education and Counseling.

HELMRATH, T. A., & Steinitz, E. M. (1978). Death of an infant: Parental grieving and the failure of social support. *The Journal of Family Practice, 6*, 785–790.

JONES, O. W., Penn, N. E., Schuchter, S., Stafford, C. A., Richards, T., Kernahan, C., Gutierrez, J., & Cherkin, P. (1984). Parental response to midtrimester therapeutic abortion following amniocentesis. *Prenatal Diagnosis, 4*, 249–259.

KESSLER, S. (1979). *Genetic counseling: Psychological dimensions.* New York: Academic Press.

LAROCHE, C., Lalinec-Michaud, M., Engelsmann, F., Fuller, N., Copp, M., McQuade-Soldatos, L., & Azima, R. (1984). Grief reactions to perinatal death—A follow-up study. *Canadian Journal of Psychiatry, 29*, 14–19.

MAGYARI, P. A., Wedehase, B. A., Ifft, R. D., & Callahan, N. P. (1987). A supportive intervention protocol for couples terminating a pregnancy for genetic reasons. *Birth Defects Original Article Series, 23*(6), 75–83.

MCNAIR, D. M., Lorr, M., Droppelman, L. F. (1971). *Manual for the Profile of Mood States.* San Diego: Educational and Industrial Testing Service.

MILNE, L. S., & Rich, O. J. (1981). Cognitive and affective aspects of the responses of pregnant women to sonography. *Maternal-Child Nursing Journal, 10*, 15–39.

NADELSON, C. C. (1978). "Normal" and "special" aspects of pregnancy: A psychological approach. In M. T. Notman and C. C. Nadelson (Eds.), *The woman patient. Vol I.* (pp. 73–86). New York: Plenum Press.

NEUGEBAUER, R., Kline, J., Susser, M., O'Connor, P., Shrout, P., Johnson, J., Skodol, A., & Wicks, J. (1992). Depressive symptoms in women in the six months following miscarriage. *American Journal of Obstetrics and Gynecology, 166*, 104–109.

OSTERWEIS, M., Solomon, F., & Green, M. (Eds.). (1984). *Bereavement: Reactions, consequences, and care*. Washington, DC: National Academy Press.

PAUL, N., & Kavanaugh, L. (Eds.). (1990). *Recommendations from the National Symposium on Genetics Services for Underserved Populations*. Washington, DC: National Center for Education in Maternal and Child Health.

PEPPERS, L. G., & Knapp, J. (1980). *Motherhood and mourning*. New York: Praeger.

RANDO, T. A. (1985). Bereaved parents: Particular difficulties, unique factors, and treatment issues. *Social Work, 30*, 19–23.

RHOADS, G. G., Jackson, L., Schlesselman, S., delaCruz, F. F., Desnick, R. J., Golbus, M. S., Ledbetter, D. H., Lubs, H. A., Mahoney, M. J., Pergament, E., Simpson, J. L., Carpenter, R. J., Elias, S., Ginsberg, N. A., Goldberg, J. D., Hobbins, J. C., Lynch, L., Shiono, P. H., Wapner, R. J., & Zachary, J. M. (1989). Safety and efficacy of transcervical chorionic villus sampling. Initial results from the U.S. collaborative study. *New England Journal of Medicine, 320*, 609–617.

ROBERTS, C. A. (1989). Research methods taught and utilized in social work. *Journal of Social Service Research, 13*, 65–86.

ROSENBLATT, P. G., & Burns, L. H. (1986). Long-term effects of perinatal loss. *Journal of Family Issues, 7*, 237–253.

ROTHMAN, B. K. (1986). *The tentative pregnancy*. New York: Penguin Books.

ROTHMAN, B. K. (1989). *Recreating Motherhood*. New York: Norton.

RUDDICK, S. (1989). *Maternal Thinking*. New York: Ballantine.

SMITH, E. M. (1973). A follow-up study of women who request abortion. *American Journal of Orthopsychiatry, 43*, 574–585.

SPANIER, G. B. (1976). Measuring dyadic adjustment: New scale for assessing the quality of marriage and similar dyads. *Journal of Marriage and Family, 38*, 15–28.

TOEDTER, L. J., Lasker, J. N., & Alhadeff, J. M. (1988). The perinatal grief scale: Development and initial validation. *American Journal of Orthopsychiatry, 58*, 435–449.

TURRINI, P. (1980). Psychological crises in normal pregnancy. In B. L. Blum (Ed.), *Psychological aspects of pregnancy, birthing, and bonding* (pp. 135–150). New York: Human Sciences Press.

VACHON, M. L. S., Sheldon, A. R., Lancee, W. J., Lyall, W. A. L., Rogers, J., & Freeman, S. J. J. (1982). Correlates of enduring stress patterns following bereavement: Social network, life situation, and personality. *Psychological Medicine, 12*, 783–788.

VIDEKA-SHERMAN, L. (1987). Research on the effect of parental bereavement: Implications for social work intervention. *Social Service Review,*
61, 102–116.

VIDEKA-SHERMAN, L., & Lieberman, M. (1985). The effects of self-help
and psychotherapy intervention on child loss: The limits of recovery.
American Journal of Orthopsychiatry, 55, 70–82.

WORTMAN, C. B., & Silver, R. C. (1989). The myths of coping with
loss. *Journal of Consulting and Clinical Psychology, 57*, 349–357.

National Institutes of Health Workshop Statement

Reproductive Genetic Testing:
Impact on Women

Reproductive genetic testing, counseling, and other genetic services can be valuable components in the reproductive health care of women and their families; they can also have negative effects on individuals, on families, and on communities. These services have the potential to increase knowledge about possible pregnancy outcomes that may occur if a woman decides to reproduce; provide reassurance during pregnancy; enhance the developing relationship between the woman, her expected child, and others; allow a woman an opportunity to choose whether to continue a pregnancy in which the expected child has a birth defect or a genetic disorder; and, if continuing, both facilitate prenatal or early infant therapy for the expected child, when possible, and prepare the family for bearing and rearing a child with a disability. Conversely, these services have the potential to increase anxiety; place excessive responsibility, blame, and guilt on a woman for her pregnancy outcome; interfere with mother-infant bonding; and disrupt relationships between a woman, family members, and her community.

The challenge is to provide each woman with an opportunity to have access to desired genetic services, in a way that will improve her control over the circumstances of her reproductive life, her pregnancies, childbearing, and parenting, within a framework that is sensitive to her needs and values and that minimizes the potential for coercion. The value that women and their families place on these services depends heavily on a mixture of psychological and ethno-cultural influences, religious and moral values, and legal and economic constraints that are unique to each woman. In addition, it may be influenced by a woman's perceptions about and past experience with people with disabilities. As a consequence, women in different circumstances may weigh the merits of reproductive genetic services quite differently.

These complex individual differences among women challenge efforts to evaluate the safety and efficacy of reproductive genetic services. To reflect the function of genetic services in reproductive health care, evaluation criteria must be client centered. That is, beyond assessment of the biological safety and technical reliability of reproductive genetic services, there should be assessment to determine whether they fulfill the roles that their clients define for them. Women may be interested in knowing to what extent reproductive genetic services can reassure, facilitate planning, and improve informed decision-making, as well as how they can limit potentially offsetting costs such as the risk for coercion, increased anxiety, and compromise of their own values. Further, it may be important to determine to what extent reproductive genetic services can be modulated to respect the needs and interests of individual women and their families. Research designed to evaluate reproductive genetic services in these terms is urgently needed.

This understanding of reproductive genetic services has several important implications that should be considered in the development of a future research agenda in this area.

1. *Reproductive genetic services should not be used to pursue "eugenic" goals but should be aimed at increasing individuals' control over their own reproductive lives. Therefore, new strategies need to be developed to evaluate the success of such services.* Reproductive genetic services must ultimately serve personal—not public—interests, in improving the overall reproductive lives of women. Whatever societal gains might be realized through the eugenic use of reproductive genetic services should be heavily outweighed by the personal needs of women and their families. The ideals of

self-determination in family matters and respect for individual differences, ideals that lie behind the client-centered view of reproductive genetic services, are jeopardized whenever the primary goal of these services becomes the prevention of the birth of individuals with a disorder or a disability. Such a goal has the potential to constrain the choices available to women and to further stigmatize those individuals affected by a particular disorder or disability. To the extent that voluntary reproductive genetic services are evaluated even indirectly in eugenic terms, societal pressures have the potential to threaten the important interests and desires of individual women and their families.

2. *Reproductive genetic services should be meticulously voluntary.* Since the primary goal of reproductive genetic services should be to enhance personal reproductive decisions, such testing should not be swept in with other "routine" or "universal" reproductive interventions, unless informed consent or refusal can be assured. Assisting women to give a fully informed consent or refusal to genetics education, testing, and counseling services is at the heart of these services. Whether reproductive genetic services are provided by genetics professionals or other health-care professionals, it is vital that these services be provided in a nonjudgmental and noncoercive manner and that the testing be carried out only after adequate education about their benefits and risks, including those beyond biology. The success of reproductive genetic services depends on their ability to effectively empower people to make knowledgeable and informed decisions. As a result, methods to evaluate the success or failure of these services should be devised with this goal in mind.

3. *Reproductive genetic services should be value sensitive.* Providers of reproductive genetic services should be particularly sensitive to individual differences and similarities—including ethnocultural differences and similarities and various constellations of beliefs, value commitments, and relationships—and should adapt their services accordingly. In particular, providers of reproductive genetic services need to be aware of their own value system, which has developed within the context and culture of the biomedical sciences, and to be aware of the language, undertones, assumptions, and values hidden within their own

professions. Training of professionals who will provide these services should include special emphasis on influences of psychological, sociodemographic, religious and moral values, and ethnocultural diversity in women's needs and interests regarding reproductive genetic testing services. The true impact that the providers' gender, race, ethnicity, class, and educational discipline have on how services are provided must be evaluated.

4. *Standards of care for reproductive genetic services should emphasize genetic information, education, and counseling rather than testing procedures alone.* To the extent that reproductive genetic services are designed to facilitate personal reproductive planning, providers of reproductive genetic testing and counseling should tailor their services to meet the needs and interests of individual women from the beginning. Extreme efforts should be made to ensure that the content of information shared regarding the disorders for which testing is carried out is comprehensive, accurate, and provided in an unbiased manner, so that a true picture of what life with such a disability may be like is presented.

Evaluation measures to determine when women know enough to have these interests met could serve to establish professional standards of care that do not drive providers to encourage testing when it is not desired. Conversely, sometimes providers do not offer reproductive genetic testing unless a woman knows enough to ask for these services. Further evaluation must be done to determine the balance which must be reached in educating women so that they have enough information about these services but do not feel pressure to utilize them when they are not desired.

5. *Social, legal, and economic constraints on reproductive genetic services should be removed.* Government and institutional policies have continued to influence legal and fiscal rules that limit the reproductive genetic testing choices that women have available to them. Research is needed to clarify such constraints and how they affect the choices and availability of services. Research is also needed to develop and test alternative models for delivery that would improve access and reduce barriers to reproductive genetic services for those women who desire them.

6. *Increasing attention focused on the development and utilization of reproductive genetic testing services may further stigmatize individ-*

uals affected by a particular disorder or disability. The values that some place on health and disabilities, what people may be told about disabilities, and even the use of certain language to describe the benefits of reproductive genetic testing have the potential to devalue the worth that individuals with disabilities have in society. Both increased sensitivity to these issues and improved communication between the biomedical and the disability communities are urgently needed in order for the true impact of these developing technologies to become known. Individuals with disabilities, who have a variety of information, experiences, and views to share, must be involved in the development and implementation of further research to be carried out in this area.

In summary, there are a number of ways that reproductive genetic services may continue to be, in many cases, less than ideal. This system of care will fail not only if providers are not informed about and sensitive to the importance of individual differences among women, but also if women themselves do not understand the complexity of making decisions about whether to utilize these services within the context of their own needs. The future of reproductive genetic testing within the context of reproductive health care of women and their families depends on research activities that are aimed at a better understanding of how best to address these challenges.

This material is in the public domain and no copyright is claimed.

This statement and the entire proceedings of this workshop were published in *Fetal Diagnosis and Therapy*, 1993, Vol. 8, Suppl. 1.

Workshop Participants

Members of the workshop were as follows: co-chairs—Elizabeth Thomson, R.N., M.S., University of Iowa, and Karen Rothenberg, J.D., M.P.A., University of Maryland School of Law; Panel members—Ruth Schwartz Cowan, Ph.D., State University of New York at Stony Brook; John Meany, Ph.D., Council of Regional Networks for Genetic Services; Jessica Davis, M.D., Cornell University; Ellen Wright Clayton, M.D.,

J.D., Vanderbilt University; Barbara Katz Rothman, Ph.D., The City University of New York; Deborah Kaplan, J.D., World Institute on Disability; Mark Evans, M.D., Wayne State University School of Medicine; Dorothy Wertz, Ph.D., Shriver Center for Mental Retardation; Rayna Rapp, Ph.D., New School of Social Research; Nancy Press, Ph.D., University of California, Los Angeles; Mary Ann Coffman, M.S., Oklahoma State Department of Health; Laurie Nsiah-Jefferson, M.P.H., New Jersey Department of Health; Ruth Faden, Ph.D., Johns Hopkins University; Patricia King, J.D., Georgetown University Law Center; Alta Charo, J.D., University of Wisconsin; Adrienne Asch, A.C.S.W., C.S.W.; Rita Beck Black, D.S.W., Columbia University; Sandra Tunis, Ph.D., University of California, San Francisco; Abby Lippman, Ph.D., McGill University; Bartha Knoppers, Ph.D., University of Montreal; Victor Penchaszadeh, M.D., Beth Israel Medical Center; Suzanne Braga, M.D., Medizinische Universitäts-Kinderklinik; Neil A. Holtzman, M.D., The Johns Hopkins Medical Institutions; Ann C. M. Smith, M.A.; Elena Gates, M.D., University of California, San Francisco; and Frederic Frigoletto, M.D., Harvard Medical School.

Workshop moderators were as follows: Jane Fullarton, M.P.A., Institute of Medicine, National Academy of Sciences; Robyn Nishimi, Ph.D., Office of Technology Assessment; Nancy Wexler, Ph.D., Columbia University and Hereditary Disease Foundation; John Fletcher, Ph.D., University of Virginia; Anita Allen, J.D., Ph.D., Georgetown University Law Center; Robin J. R. Blatt, M.P.H., R.N., Massachusetts Department of Public Health; Maurice J. Mahoney, M.D., Yale University School of Medicine; and Elsa Gomez, Ph.D., Pan American World Health Organization.

Cosponsors were the National Institute of Child Health and Human Development, National Center for Human Genome Research, National Center for Nursing Research, and the Office of Research on Women's Health.

RITA BECK BLACK, M.S., D.S.W., is associate professor at the Columbia University School of Social Work and assistant project director of the Maternal and Child Health Training Grant. She has trained in both social work and genetic counseling, and her research and publications have centered on the psychosocial dimensions of genetic and reproductive technologies. She is co-author of *Social Work and Genetics: A Guide for Practice*.

CAROLE H. BROWNER, Ph.D., M.P.H., is professor in the Department of Psychiatry and Bio-behavior Sciences and the Department of Anthropology at UCLA. She is a medical anthropologist with more than fifteen years' experience in Colombia, Mexico, and the Unites States on issues concerning women's reproductive health and health care decision-making. She has published widely and is now working on a monograph on the politics of reproduction for Cambridge University Press.

R. ALTA CHARO, J.D., is assistant professor of law and medical ethics at the Schools of Law and Medicine at the University of Wisconsin. She specializes in the politics of biology and human reproduction. Recent writings have appeared in the *Texas Journal of Women and the Law* and the *St. Louis University Law Review*.

ELLEN WRIGHT CLAYTON, M.D., J.D., is assistant professor of law and of pediatrics at Vanderbilt University and is a Charles E. Culpeper Foundation Scholar in Medical Humanities. She has a longstanding interest in the implications of reproductive genetic technologies. Her research has also included studies of informed consent, the doctor–patient relationship, and factors that lead patients to sue their physicians. She has published widely in the legal, medical, and ethics literature.

RUTH SCHWARTZ COWAN, Ph.D., is professor of history at the State University of New York, Stony Brook. She is a historian of science, currently writing a history of prenatal diagnosis. She also writes and teaches in the fields of women's history and the history of technology.

RUTH FADEN, Ph.D., M.P.H., is director of the Program in Law, Ethics, and Health at Johns Hopkins University, and she is senior research scholar at the Kennedy Institute of Ethics at Georgetown University. Her primary area of scholarship is in ethics and health policy, with a particular focus on issues affecting women and children.

ELENA A. GATES, M.D., is associate clinical professor in the Department of Obstetrics, Gynecology, and Reproductive Sciences at the University of California, San Francisco. In addition to her clinical work, she is active in the area of medical ethics, particularly as it applies to reproductive medicine. Her recent work has focused on the ethical considerations concerning prenatal genetic testing and fetal treatment.

DEBORAH KAPLAN, J.D., is an attorney with a disability who focuses on disability public policy. She is vice president of the World Institute on Disability, and director of its Division on Technology Policy.

PATRICIA A. KING, J.D., is professor of law at the Georgetown University Law Center, and her expertise is in the study of law, medicine, ethics, and public policy. She is coauthor of *Cases and Materials on Law, Science, and Medicine* and has published widely in the area of reproductive ethics. She has served on numerous national and bioethics commissions and groups including the Ethical, Legal, and Social Implications (ELSI) working group of the Human Genome Project.

ABBY LIPPMAN, Ph.D., is professor of epidemiology and biostatistics at McGill University, Montreal, and she chairs the Human Genetics Committee of the Council for Responsible Genetics, Cambridge, MA. In her research and activism she focuses on the application of genetics from a feminist perspective, emphasizing the increasing geneticization of health and illness and the biopolitics of biomedicine. She has published widely in both the professional and lay literature.

MARY B. MAHOWALD, Ph.D., is professor at the Pritzker School of Medicine and MacLean Center for Clinical Medical Ethics, University of Chicago. She taught philosophy for fifteen years before moving to a hospital and medical school complex in 1982. Her most recent book, *Women and Children in Health Care: An Unequal Majority*, elaborates her philosophical orientation and emphasis.

LAURIE NSIAH-JEFFERSON, M.P.H., is a research scientist for the New Jersey State Department of Health. She has expertise in the areas of reproductive health issues as they relate to low-income women and women of color and has worked with many agencies and programs on issues relating to perinatal addictions, AIDS, maternal and child health, and reproductive genetic testing. She has published in such journals as *Fetal Diagnosis and Therapy* and the *Women's Rights Law Reporter*, as well as in the books *Women, Health, and Technology: Perspectives & Prescriptions* and *Reproductive Laws for the 1990s*.

NANCY ANNE PRESS, Ph.D., is a medical anthropologist in the psychiatry department at UCLA. Her major areas of interest are women and health, bioethics, and genetics. She has presented lectures and published a number of papers on these issues. She is a member of the advisory board for the University of Washington's Ethical Paradigms in Genetics Project, and she is on the Clinical Ethics Committee at UCLA.

RAYNA RAPP, Ph.D., is professor of anthropology and chair of gender studies and feminist theory at the New School for Social Research. She is currently completing a book on the social impact and cultural meaning of prenatal diagnosis based on anthropological field work in New York City. She has been active in the movement for women's studies and for reproductive rights for over twenty years, and has published widely.

KAREN H. ROTHENBERG, J.D., M.P.A., is the Marjorie Cook professor of law and director of the law and health care program at the University of Maryland School of Law. She specializes in health law particularly in the area of women's health and has published articles in the *New England Journal of Medicine*; *Law, Medicine, and Health Care*; and numerous law reviews. She is currently president of the American Society of Law, Medicine, and Ethics.

BARBARA KATZ ROTHMAN, Ph.D., is professor of sociology at the Baruch College and the Graduate Center of the City University of New York. Her major work on women and reproductive testing, *The Tentative Pregnancy: How Amniocentesis Changes the Experience of Motherhood*, has also been published in Great Britain and in Germany. Her other books include *Recreating Motherhood* and *In Labor: Women and Power in the Birthplace*, and she edited *The Encyclopedia of Childbearing*.

ELIZABETH J. THOMSON, M.S., R.N., is coordinator of genetics services research in the Ethical, Legal, and Social Implications Branch of the National Center for Human Genome Research. She is board certified in genetic counseling by the American Board of Medical Genetics and has also been actively involved in a number of nursing and genetics organizations, including cofounding the Genetics Nurse Network, which became the International Society of Nurses in Genetics. In addition, she has published papers and given presentations on genetics, birth defects, nurses' roles in providing genetic services, and genetic counseling.

Women and Health Series

Rima D. Apple and Janet Golden, Editors

The series examines the social and cultural construction of
health practices and policies, focusing on women as subjects
and objects of medical theory, health services, and policy
formulation.

*The Selling of Contraception: The Dalkon Shield Case, Sexuality,
and Women's Autonomy*
Nicole J. Grant

*And Sin No More: Social Policy and Unwed Mothers in Cleveland,
1855–1990*
Marian J. Morton